Introduction

This is the 1st edition of a "pathway" using the A to Z format.

It encompasses all the structures involved in the digestion of food from the beginning to end, which is why all the structures from lips to buttocks have been included. They all play a role. Remember when the anus shuts down – nothing works: the brain cannot think; the eyes cannot see; the legs cannot run... and this means... do not forget ALL the factors.

I hope it has been successful – Please let me know what you think.

The A to Zs may be viewed on 2 sites - www.amandasatoz.com and http://www.aspenpharma.com.au/atlas/student.htm

Feedback can be left at

medicalamanda@gmail.com

Acknowledgement

Thank you Aspenpharmacare Australia for your support and assistance in this valuable project, particularly Greg Lan, Rob Koster, Richard Clement, Peter Penn, Phill Ryman and Quentin and everyone who provided valuable feedback.

Dedication

To all those people out there who have an interest in their DIGESTIVE SYSTEM from the entrance to the exit. Those dieting and those not, those who cook and those who don't, those health conscious and those not, those with fussy palates and those without – WE ALL EAT!!!

How to use this book

The format of this A to Z book has been maintained as in the last edition – the beginning has overviews and then the sections of the Digestive tract = DT are broken up and listed alphabetically and cross referenced for ease of data retrieval. The book is its own index in each section.

As with all the A to Z books - think of it and then find it alphabetically.

Cross referencing in the index is in the usual manner i.e. *see* for go to and *see also* for additional images listed under that heading, and this book is cross-referenced with all the other *A to Zs*.

Thank you

A. L. Neill

BSc MSc MBBS PhD FACBS

ISBN 978 1 921930 00 3

T0319299

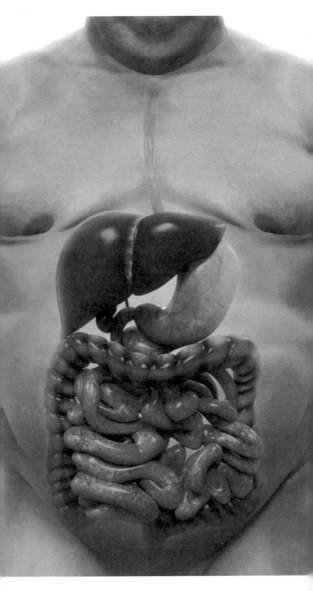

Table of contents

Abbreviations

a	= artery	EAM	= external acoustic meatus
aa	= anastomosis (ses)	EAS	= external anal sphincter
ACF	= anterior cranial fossa	EC	= extracellular (outside the cell)
adj.	= adjective		
aka	= also known as	ext.	= extensor (as in muscle to extend across a joint)
alt.	= alternative		
ANS	= autonomic nervous system	GALT	= gut associated lymphoid tissue
ant.	= anterior	GB	= gall bladder
art.	= articulation (joint w/o the additional support structures)	gld	= gland
		GIT	= gastro-intestinal tract
		Gk.	= Greek
AS	= Alternative Spelling, generally referring to the diff. b/n British & American spelling	H	= hormone
		HP	= high pressure
		I	= insertion
		IBD	= inflammatory bowel disease
ASIS	= anterior superior iliac spine (of hip bone)		
		IAS	= internal anal sphincter
bc	= because	jt(s)	= joints = articulations
BF	= blood flow	l	= lymphatic
BM	= basement membrane	L	= lumbar / left
b/n	= between	LI	= large intestine
br	= branch	lig	= ligament
BS	= Blood Supply	LP	= lumbar plexus/lamina proporia/
CC	= cerebral cortex		
c.f.	= compared to	LP	= Low pressure
CN	= cranial nerve	Lt.	= Latin
CNS	= central nervous system	m	= muscle
Co	= coccygeal	MCL	= mid clavicular line
CP	= cervical plexus	med.	= medial
collat.	= collateral	MM	= mucous membrane
Cr	= cranial	N (s)	= nerve(s)
CT	= connective tissue	NAD	= normal (size, shape)
DT	= digestive tract	NAD	= no abnormality detected
diff.	= difference(s)	NR	= nerve root origin
dist.	= distal	NS	= nervous supply / nerve system
DM	= dura mater		
Duo	= duodenum	NT	= nervous tissue
e.g.	= example		

nv	= neurovascular bundle
O	= origin
P	= pressure
PaNS	= parasympathetic nervous system
ParaNs	= parasympathetic nerves ± fibres
pl.	= plural
PN	= peripheral nerve
post.	= posterior
proc.	= process
prox.	= proximal
R	= right / resistance
SC	= spinal cord
SCM	= sternocleidomastoid muscle
SI	= small intestine
sing.	= singular
SN	= spinal nerve
SP	= spinous process / sacral plexus
SS	= signs and symptoms
subcut	= subcutaneous (just under the skin)
supf	= superficial
SyNS	= sympathetic nervous system
T	= TEST / thoracic
TC	= Transverse colon
TMJ	= temporomandibular joint
Tx	= therapy / treatment
UC	= ulcerative colitis
UL	= upper limb, arm
V	= vertebra / vein
VB	= vertebral body
VC	= vertebral column
WM	= white matter
w/n	= within

w/o	= without
wrt	= with respect to
&	= and
∩	= intersection with

Common terms in the Study and Examination of the Digestive Tract.

Ablation
the removal of part of the body, generally a bony part, most commonly the teeth.

Additus
opening /entrance.

Adenoid
gland.

Ala
a wing, hence a wing-like process as in the Ethmoid bone *pl.-alae.*

Alveolus
air filled bone - tooth socket *adj.- alveolar* (as in air filled bone in the maxilla)

Annulus fibrosis
the peripheral fibrous ring around the intervertebral disc.

Ansa
loop-like structure

Aperture
an opening or space between bones or within a bone.

Areola
small, open spaces as in the areolar part of the axilla may lead or develop into sinuses.

Basiocranium
bones of the base of the skull

Bite
to bring the upper and lower jaws together - *noun the Bite - the examination of the closed jaws see Occlusion.*

Buccal
pertaining to the cheek

Canal
tunnel / extended foramen as in the carotid canal at the base of the skull adj. - canular (canicular - small canal).

Carotid
to put to sleep; compression of the common or internal carotid artery causes coma. This refers to bony points related to the Carotid vessels.

Cavity
an open area or sinus within a bone or formed by two or more bones *(adj. - cavernous)*, may be used interchangeably with fossa. A Cavity tends to be more enclosed, a fossa a shallower bowl-like space (Orbital fossa - Orbital cavity).

Cementum
fibres often w/in the periodontal membrane around the teeth attaching them to the socket.

Cephalic
pertaining to the head

Chief cells
produce pesinogen, inactive form of pepsin the enzymewhich digests protein - converts the active form in an acid environment

Chyme
the liquid which leaves the stomach after it has been digested

Colitis
inflammation of the colon

Colon
term used interchangeably with Large intestine (LI) but actually only consisting of 4 parts - the ascending + transverse + descending + sigmoid colons – not including the caecum or appendix which are usually included in the LI.

Concha
a shell shaped bone as in the ear or nose. *(pl. - conchae adj. - conchoid)* old term for this turbinate.

Constipation
difficult, incomplete evacuation of the faecal material from the colon.

Constrictor
to squeeze

Cornu
a horn (as in the Hyoid)

Corona — a crown. *adj. - coronary, coronoid or coronal;* hence a coronal plane is parallel to the main arch of a crown which passes from ear to ear (c.f. coronal suture).

Cranium — the cranium of the skull comprises all of the bones of the skull except for the mandible.

Crest — a prominent sharp thin ridge of bone formed by the attachment of muscles particularly powerful ones e.g. Temporalis forming the Sagittal crest.

Cribiform/Ethmoid — a sieve or bone with small sieve-like holes.

Cricoid — a ring

-crine — **to secrete**

Cutus — skin - hence cutaneous branches refers to the nerves supplying the skin and adnexae.

Dens — a tooth hence dentine and dental relating to teeth, denticulate having tooth-like projections *adj. - dentate* also refers to a serrated edge as in the dentate line b/n anus and rectum.

Depression — a concavity on a surface.

Dentine (aka) dentin — ivory - like substance forming the bulk of the tooth beneath the enamel.

Diarrhoea AS Diarrhea — frequent evacuation of watery faecal material - generally pathological.

Distal — further away from the axial skeleton (opposite of Proximal)

Dorsi — back

Edentulous — without teeth

Eminence — a smooth projection or elevation on a bone as in iliopubic eminence.

Endocrine — secretion of a substance from cells directly to the BS w/o a duct

Enteritis — inflammation of the bowel, generally the SI

Entero- — **pertaining to the bowel**

Exocrine — secretion of substances from cells via ducts as in exocrine glands generally into a lumen

Facet — A face, a small bony surface (occlusal facet on the chewing surfaces of the teeth) seen in planar joints.

Facies — Face or appearance may be used to designate a number of facial expressions or systemic conditions eg steroid facies.

Fascia — a sheet of fibrous CT which surrounds muscles, organs and regions - often supporting their BS & NS.

Fasciule — fasces / fasicules / bundles / small bundles

Fauces — jaws or throat

Fissure — a narrow slit or gap from cleft.

Flexure — a fixed bend generally due to a tether by lig or mesentery to the peritoneal wall as in the Hepatic flexure of the LI

Foramen — a natural hole in a bone usually for the transmission of blood vessels and/or nerves.*(pl. foramina).*

Fossa	a pit, depression, or concavity, on a bone, or formed from several bones as in temporomandibular fossa. Shallower and more like a "bowl" than a cavity.
Fovea	a small pit (usually smaller than a fossa)- as in the fovea of the occlusal surface of the molar tooth.
GALT	a general term for all the lymphoid tissue associated with the GIT
Gastric	belly (as in the belly of a muscle)
Gingiva	gum
Glottis	pertaining to the vocal cords and structures involved in the production of the voice.
Gomphosis	joint b/n the roots of the teeth and the jaw bones *pl. - gomphoses*
Groove	long pit or furrow
Haematemesis	blood in vomit
Haematochezia	bright red clots of blood in the stools
Hamus	a hook hence the term used for bones which "hook around other bones or where other structures are able to attach by hooking - hamulus = a small hook.
Hyoid	U-shaped
Ileitis	inflammation of the ileum
Incisura	a notch.
Inferior	under
Inter	between
Intra	within
Intracrine	secretion in a cell which acts internally on actions in that cell.
Intracrine Introitus	an orifice or point of entry to a cavity or space.
Labial	pertaining to the lips.
Lacerum	something lacerated, mangled or torn e.g. foramen lacerum small sharp hole at the base of the skull often ripping.
Lacrimal	related to tears and tear drops. *(noun - lacrima).*
Lamina	a plate as in the lamina of the vertebra, a plate of bone connecting the vertical and transverse spines *(pl. - laminae).*
Levator	to raise
Ligament	A ligament is a tie or a connection. Originally *sing.- igamentum pl.- ligamenta.*
Linea	a line as in the nuchal lines of the Occitipum.
Lingual	pertaining to the tongue
Malar	cheek
Malleus	hammer (as in the ear ossicle)
Malocclusion	misalignment of the teeth as in over-bite or under-bite
Mandible	from the verb to chew, hence, the movable lower jaw; *adj. - mandibular.*
Masseter	to chew
Mastoid	a breast or teat shape - mastoid process of the Temporal bone.

Maxilla	the jaw-bone; now used only for the upper jaw; *adj. - maxillary.*
Meatus	a short passage; *adj. - meatal* as in EAM connecting the outer ear with the middle ear.
Mental	relating to the chin (**mentum = chin <u>not</u> mens = mind).**
Mesial	along the dental arch in the direction of the medial plane anteriorly (opposite to distal).
Modiolus	hub or cental core used in the face to indicate that fibrous hub at the edge of the mouth for the insertion of a number of muscles /used in the ear to indicate the centre of the spongy bone of the cochlea tubes.
Mucosa	tissue in the GIT immediately beneath the epithelial lining.
Mucus	substance excreted by Mucous glands to lubricate food or protect mucosal surfaces - i.e. *noun - mucus/ adj. - mucous, mucoid.*
Muscularis Mucosa	term for the muscle layer in the mucosa separating the mucosa from the submucosa.
Naris	nostrils *pl. - nares*
Notch	an indentation in the margin of a structure.
Nucha	the nape or back of the neck *adj. - nuchal.*
Occulus	an eye
Odontoid	relating to teeth, toothlike *see Dens*
Omo	shoulder
Orbit	a circle; the name given to the bony socket in which the eyeball rotates; *adj. - orbital.*
Orifice	an opening.
Palate	a roof *adj. palatal or palatine.*
Papilla	outpouching – point generally with an opening as in the duodenal papilla; *pl. - papillae.*
Parietal	pertaining to the outer wall of a cavity from paries, a wall.
Parotid	pertaining to a region beside or near the ear.
Pars	a part of
Pecten	a comb.
Perikymata	transverse ridges and the grooves on the surfaces of teeth.
Periodontum	CT membrane surrounding the tooth to allow for support and cushioning of tooth movements with mastication.
Periosteum	layer of fascial tissue, CT on the outside of compact bone not present on articular. (joint) surfaces.
Peristalsis	the automatic coordinated contraction & relaxation of the GIT smooth muscle triggered by the presence of a food bolus & propagated by the internal NS of the GIT the Auerbach & Myenteric plexi – directing food in one direction
Petrous	pertaining to a rock / rocky / stoney *adj. - petrosal*
Plica (e)	fold(s) generally fixed folds as found in the SI.

Process	a general term describing any marked projection or prominence as in the mandibular process.
Proximal	closer to the axial skeleton (opposite of distal).
Raphe	line of joint b/n two halves, generally of bone or muscles for e.g. a fibrous raphe in the tongue allowing for muscle insertion.
Recess	a secluded area or pocket; a small cavity set apart from a main cavity.
Rectus	straight - erect
rhino-	**pertaining to the nose**
Ridge	elevated bony growth often roughened.
Rotundum	round
Ruga (e)	folds – generally more mobile and less structured than Plicae
Sagittal	an arrow, the sagittal suture is notched posteriorly, making it look like an arrow by the lambdoid sutures. *See Anatomical planes.*
Sclerosis	hard
Septum	a division
Sinus	a space usually w/n a bone lined with mm, such as the frontal and maxillary sinuses in the head, (also, a space usually w/in a bone, may contain air, blood or mucous. *adj.- sinusoid* Sinusoid capillaries are found in the liver and wide enough to have cellular elements pass into the lumen.
Skull	the skull refers to all of the bones that comprise the head.
Spine	a thorn *adj. - spinous,* descriptive of a sharp, slender process/protrusion.
Sphincter	ring of muscle around a tube or opening.
Splanchocranium	the splanchocranium refers to the facial bones of the skull.
-stoma	**to do with the mouth**
Subcutaneous	under the skin
Submucosa	layer common to all the gut layers deep to the mucosa
Sulcus	long wide groove often due to a BV indentation.
Suture	the saw-like edge of a cranial bone that serves as jt b/n bones of the skull.
Sulcus	furrow
Superior	above
Syn	**means together i.e. the close proximity of or fusion of two structures**
Temporal	refers to time and the fact that grey hair (marking the passage of time) often appears first at the site of the Temporal bone.
Tendon	a tie or cord of collagen fibres connecting muscle with bone (as opposed to articular ligaments which connect bone with bone).
Tenesmus	an urgent but ineffectual desire to constantly defaecate or urinate seen in UC
Tensor	to stretch
Tonsil	little pole

Trachea	rough
Transverse	to go across
Tuberosity	a large rounded process or eminence, a swelling or large rough prominence often associated with a tendon or ligament attachment.
Turbinate	a child's spinning top, hence shaped like a top. An old term for the nasal conchae.
Uvula	little grape
Vagina	a sheath; hence, invagination is the acquisition of a sheath by pushing inwards into a structure, and evagination is similar but produced by pushing outwards *adj. - vaginal.*
Vomer	plough
Wormian bone	extrasutural bone in the skull.
Xerostomia	dry mouth
Zygal	H - shaped
Zygoma	a yoke, hence, the bone joining the maxillary, frontal, temporal & sphenoid bones *adj. - zygomatic.*

Anatomical planes and Anatomical positions

A = Anterior Aspect from the front = or / Posterior Aspect from the back. Used interchangeably with ventral and dorsal respectively

B = Lateral Aspect from either side

C = Transverse / Horizontal plane

D = Midsagittal plane = Median plane; trunk moving away from this plane = lateral flexion or lateral movement
plane medial movement;
limbs moving away from this direction = abduction
limbs moving closer to this plane = adduction
Note parasagittal plane / sagittal plane - indicates planes in the same direction but other than in the middle

E = Coronal plane

F = Median

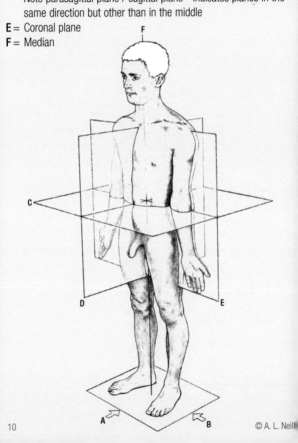

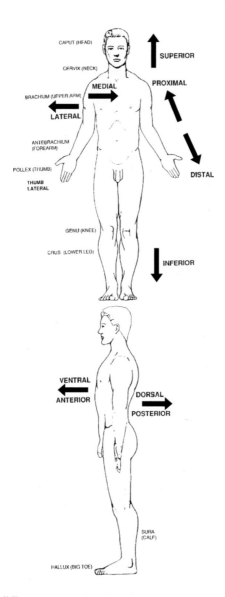

Notes...

The Digestive Tract – Overviews

Digestive Tract (DT) overview

Anterior

Definition: the DT consists of the tunnel from mouth to anus. It has a number of glands and organs which feed into it and are necessary for its function. It is a 3D structure.

1 Nasal septum dividing the nasal cavity & cartilages
2 Oral cavity
3 Tongue
4 Salivary glands s = sublingual & submandibular
  p = parotid
5 Trachea
6 Stomach (semi-concealed by the liver)
7 Spleen
8 Pancreas (retroperitoneal)
9 LI a = ascending d = descending s = sigmoid
  t = transverse
10 SI i = ileum j = jejunum
11 Rectum
12 Anus
13 Appendix
14 Gall bladder
15 Duodenum
16 Liver
17 Oesophagus
18 Pharynx
19 Phayngeal sphincters superior / middle / inferior
20 sulcus for the IVC
21 renal impression on the Liver
22 Taeni coli + haustrations
23 Thyroid cartilage
24 Buccinator with parotid duct protruding

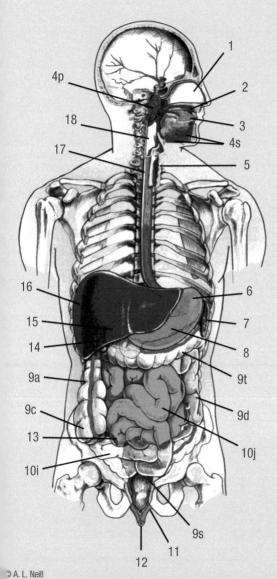

Digestive Tract overview

Posterior

Definition: the DT consists of the tunnel from mouth to anus, it has a number of glands and organs which feed into it and are necessary for its function. It is a 3D structure.

1 Nasal septum dividing the nasal cavity & cartilages
2 Oral cavity
3 Tongue
4 Salivary glands s = sublingual & submandibular
 p = parotid
5 Trachea
6 Stomach (semi-concealed by the liver)
7 Spleen
8 Pancreas (retroperitoneal)
9 LI a = ascending d = descending s = sigmoid
 t = transverse
10 SI i = ileum j = jejunum
11 Rectum
12 Anus
13 Appendix
14 Gall bladder
15 Duodenum
16 Liver
17 Oesophagus
18 Pharynx
19 Phayngeal sphincters superior / middle / inferior
20 sulcus for the IVC
21 renal impression on the Liver
22 Taeni coli + haustrations
23 Thyroid cartilage
24 Buccinator with parotid duct protruding

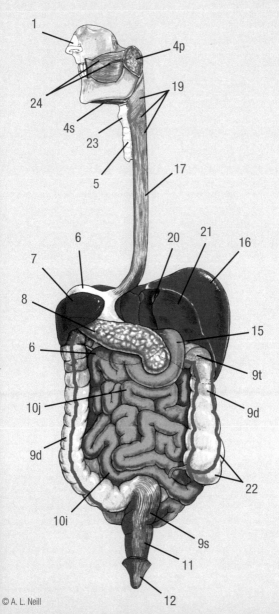

© A. L. Neill

Mouth – Oral Cavity

Open mouth – anterior view – looking into the oral cavity

Description: The oral cavity is the first point of the DT where food enters. It is masticated / pulverized & lubricated – and exposed to the ring of immune defense, the tonsils and tonsilar tissue. These form a rim at the back of the throat. The saliva commences food breakdown and water soluble elements including alcohol are directly absorbed, through the oral mucosa.

1 Labial frenulum i = inf / s = superior

2 Incisive papilla

3 Palatine rugae = transverse palatine plicae

4 Orbicularis oris large circle of muscle around the lips

5 Subcutaneous fat – in the cheek

6 Buccal fold

7 Pterygomandibular fold (+ retromalar trigone & retromolar fossa)

8 Dorsum of the tongue + median lingual sulcus

9 Superficial muscles in the facial fascia – muscles of expression*

10 Lingual fold

11 Lips (labia) & gums (gingiva) – i = inf / s = superior

12 Oropharynx – posterior wall

13 Palatoglossal arch (fold)

14 Palatine tonsil

15 Palatopharyngeal fold

16 Uvula – pendulous extension of the soft palate

17 Palates – hard & soft

18 Labial fold = vestibular oral fold

*for more details of the bones & muscles see the A to Z of the Head & Neck bones & muscles

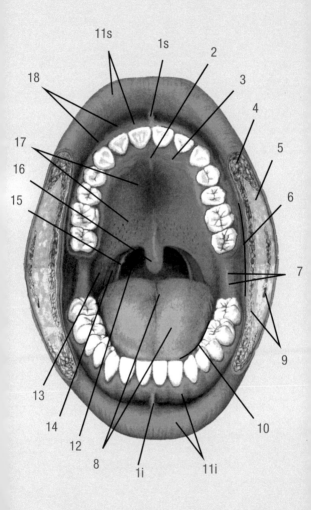

Roof of the Mouth – Palates (hard + soft)

Inferior view - looking up onto the roof of the mouth

Description: The hard palate is formed by the fusion of the 2 Maxilla bones + 2 Palatine bones*; the soft palate by the muscles and tissues of the region along with part of the ring of lymphoid tissues (tonsils) which surround the entrance to the pharynx.

1 Rugae on the hard palate – made up of hard mucosal tissue
2 Mucous glands under the epithelial lining
3 Muscles of the lips – eg Orbicularis oris + fat
4 Buccinator
5 Insertion raphe
6 Superior pharyngeal constrictor
7 Tonsil (note this is much larger and quite visible in a child and in infections)
8 Entrance to oral pharynx
9 Uvula = pendulous extension of the soft palate
10 Tongue
11 Muscles of the soft palate – involved in snoring
12 Palatoglossus
13 Palatopharyngeus
14 Palatine bone
15 Lesser palatine Ns – emerging from the lesser pharyngeal fossa
16 Greater palatine Ns and BVs – emerging from the greater palatine fossa
17 Maxilla inf surface
18 Nasopalatine Ns & BVs emerging from the Alveolare (not shown)

for details of the bones & muscles see the A to Z of the Head & Neck bones & muscles

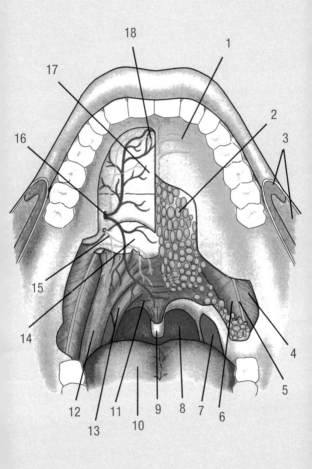

Floor of the Mouth – Salivary Glands

Superior view – tongue and mucosa removed - looking down onto the floor of the mouth

Description: The floor of the mouth is made up of muscles which lift and lower with swallowing, helping to position food to the back of the mouth and force it into the pharynx. 2 of the 3 salivary glands lie on this floor.

1 Coronoid process – attachment site of Temporalis

2 Mandibular foramen – site of entry of inf. alveolar N br of the Mandibular N – innervates all the lower teeth & ½ the tongue and lip

3 Lingual lip – on the side of the foramen

4 Angle of the jaw

5 Mylohyoid m

6 Stylohyoid m

7 Geniohyoid m

8 Hyoid bone

9 Submandibular duct

10 Submandibular gld

11 Condylar process – articulation with the TMJ

12 Lingual N – sensation of the gums & tongue – including taste

13 Sublingual gld

14 Mandibular art & N

for details of the bones, muscles & Nerves see the A to Z of the Head & Neck bones & muscles & The A to Z of Peripheral Ns

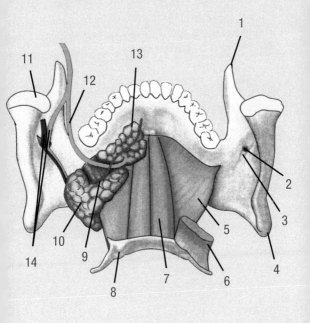

Mouth – Muscles of the oral area

Medial view – looking into the interior of the L side

Description: Muscles of the face are often inserted into the deep fascia and move the facial walls. Many of those affecting the lips and mouth opening insert into a common structure the Modiolus. There is a crossover b/n muscles of the Face, the Jaw, the Palate and the Pharynx - to facilitate a smooth path from the lips to the throat and continue the swallowing process.

note this whole surface is covered with mucosa

1 Orbicularis oris large circle of muscle around the lips
   i = labii inferioris
   L = labial part
   m = marginal part
   s = labii superioris

2 Mandible

3 Mylohyoid m

4 Platysma m

5 Modiolus

6 Palatoglossus m

7 Medial pterygoid m

8 Buccinator m

9 Buccopharyngeal part of the Superior pharyngeal constrictor m

10 Uvula – pendulous extension of the soft palate

11 Insertion raphe

12 Palate h = hard / s = soft

13 palate mucosa

14 papilla of the parotid gland

for more details of the bones & muscles see the A to Z of the Head & Neck bones & muscles

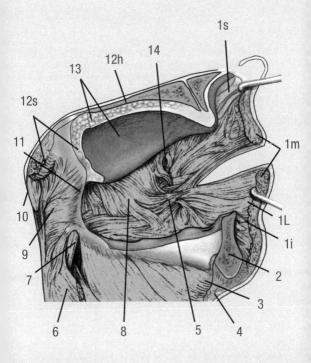

1s

14

12h

13

1m

12s

11

1L

10

1i

9

2

7

3

6   8   5   4

JAWS
Blood Supply – arterial

Schematic lateral view showing the arterial supply of the Mandible, Maxilla and the Teeth

Description: Teeth play a major role in the digestive process – from the inability to eat certain foods w/o them to the development of disease through defects in them. This diagram shows the intimate relationship b/n arteries of the teeth and other oral structures.

1 Middle meningeal a
  f = frontal br
  p = parietal br
  t = tympanic br
2 Sphenopalantine a
3 Infraorbital a
4 Post. sup. alveolar a
5 Descending palatine a
6 Buccal a
7 Pterygoid a
8 Masserteric a
9 Deep temporal a
10 Mylohyoid a
11 Tonsillar a
12 Dental a
13 Facial a
14 Mental a
15 Carotid a   c = common / e = external / i = internal
16 Ascending palatine a
17 Ascending pharyngeal a
18 Auricular a
19 Post. meningeal a
20 Maxillary a
21 Inf. alveolar a

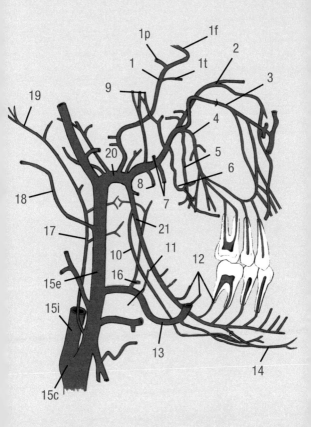

JAWS
Nerve Supply

Schematic: lateral view showing the innervation of the Mandible, Maxilla and the Teeth

Description: Teeth play a major role in the digestive process – from the inability to eat certain foods w/o them to the development of disease through defects in them.

1 Ant. sup. alveolar Ns
2 Mental N
3 Inf. dental brs
4 Inf alveolar N
5 Mylohyoid N
6 Masseteric N
7 Lingual N
8 Mandibular N - CN V_3
9 Trigeminal N - CN V
10 Ophthalmic N - CN V_1
11 Maxillary N - CN V_2
12 Zygomatic N
13 post. sup. alveolar N
14 Middle sup. alveolar N
15 Infraorbital N

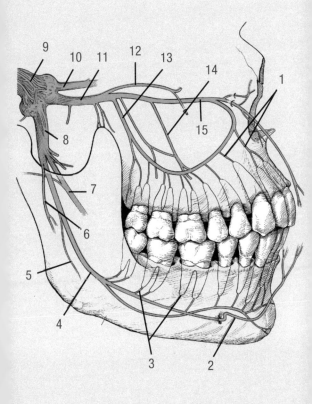

© A. L. Neill

JAWS
Blood Supply – venous

Schematic lateral view -
showing the venous supply of the Mandible, Maxilla and the teeth

Description: The venous system of the Head & Neck has deep plexi associated with the central BS and so infections of the mouth, teeth or anywhere on the face may be carried to the contents of the cranial cavity.

1 Infraorbital v
2 Ant. sup. alveolar v
3 Dental v
4 Peridental v
5 Maxillary cuspid v
6 Facial v
7 Mandibular cuspid v
8 Mental foramen
9 Mental v
10 Submental v
11 Mylohyoid v
12 Retromandibular v
13 Inf. alveolar v
14 Deep facial v
15 Maxillary v
16 Pterygoid venous plexus
17 Post. superior alveolar v

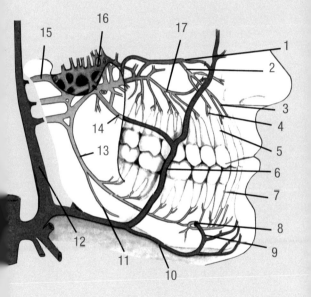

Throat – overview

Lateral view – with tissues cut away to show their relationships.

Description: The throat is the passage through which everything must pass: air, food & liquids. It is the junction point of the oral and nasal passages, separating the air from the solid material via the epiglottis. It also connects with the ears via their drainage channels the Eustachian tubes. The Pharnyx – a muscular tube from the base of the skull to the oesophagus is its main component.

1 Hard palate
2 Glossopharyngeal N
3 Epiglottis
4 Cricoid cartilage = Adams apple
5 Trachea = air passage
6 Oesophagus = food passage
7 Eustachain tube = auditory tube
8 Soft Palate

A = nasal cavity
B = oral cavity
C = nasaopharynx
D = oropharynx
E = laryngopharnyx
C + D + E = pharynx

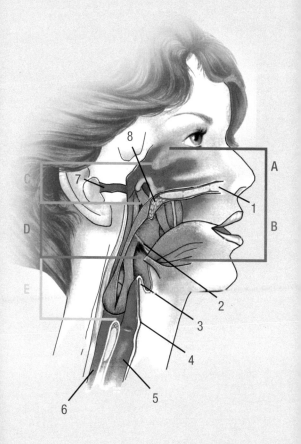

Tonsils – in situ

Lateral view - with tissues cut away to show their relationships
Mouth of a child

Description: The tonsils form a defense ring around air and food pathways. Even though they play a role in the defense of substances passing through – in infected states – tonsilitis -they swell and compromise access of air and food to the body.

1   Nasopharynx

2   Hard Palate

3   Oropharynx

4   Tongue

5   Lingual tonsil – on the root of the tongue

6   Epiglottis – Vallecula

7   Palatine tonsil

8   Pharyngeal folds/arches – for funnelling food into the oesophagus

9   Adenoids = Pharyngeal tonsils

10 Nasopharynx

As the mouth – jaw increases in size so does the pharynx – and swollen tonsils are not as obstructive to food and air.

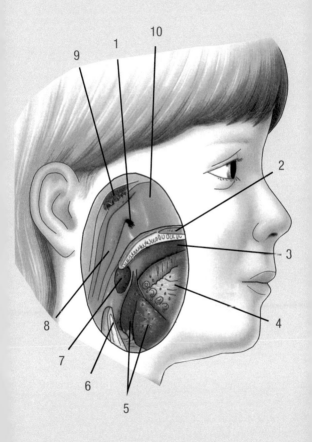

Gastro-Intestinal Tract = GIT overview
schema

Description: The GIT is a long muscular tube consisting of several parts involved the breakup and digestion of food. The GIT is 5m (20ft) long (9m (30ft) w/o muscle tone). It is may be divided into the upper GIT & the lower GIT, or the foregut, midgut and hindgut embryologically.

1 Oesophagus (10-14cm) – transport tube from the mouth to the stomach

2 Oesophagal Sphincter#

3 Stomach– acidic environment (pH1-4) to digest food and kill bacteria

4 Pyloric sphincter - dividing the stomach & the duodenum (smooth muscle) regulating food entrance into the SI

5 Duodenum – 25cm long - site of entrance of bile and pancreatic enzymes

6 Jejunum 2/5 of the total length of the SI – main site of absorption of nutrients

7 Ileum 3/5 of the SI

6 + 7 = SI – transition b/n 6 and 7 is gradual

8 ileocaecal junction – separating the SI and the LI via the ileocaecal valve, site of B12 and bile absorption

9 Veriform appendix – function? Unknown

10 Caecum – storage sac of the LI

11 Colon – H = Haustra / Haustrations = outpouchings in the wall where the longitudinal muscle is discontinuous T = taeni coli – the discontinuous outer smooth muscle layer of the LI – storage site – minimal digestion – 4 parts – site of storage and faecal concentration.

Not a true sphincter – rather a functioning "physiological" sphincter

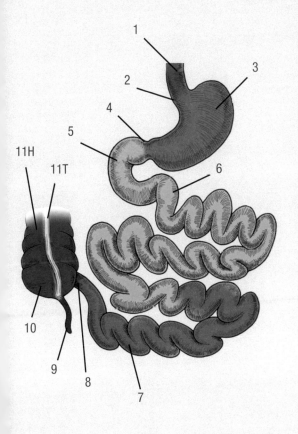

GIT overview – Blood Supply
Arterial supply – Abdominal Aorta

Anterior view – schema

The abdominal aorta is bound superiorly by the diaphragm and terminates as the common iliac arteries at the level of L5. The visceral branches are unpaired LP vessels with slow BF controlled by sphincters at their entrance, and have large networks of BVs

1-3 are Parietal paired branches

1   Inferior Phrenic a

2   Lumbar a from L1-4

3   Common iliac a

4 is an unpaired parietal branch

4   Median sacral a

5-7 are unpaired Visceral branches – and part of the portal system

5   Coeliac trunk – supplies the base of the oesophagus to the duodenum

6   Superior mesenteric a – supplies to the – mid TC

7   Inferior mesenteric a – supplies – to the rectum

8-9 are Visceral paired branches

8   Renal a

8a Adrenal a

9   Gonadal a (ovarian ♀ / testicular ♂)

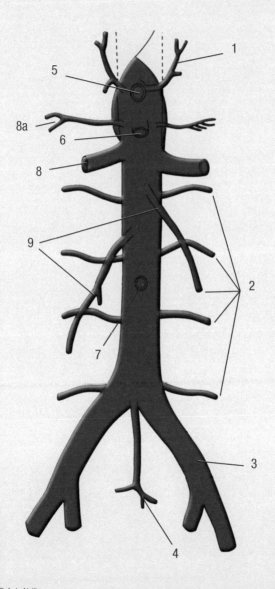

GIT overview – Blood Supply
Venous supply

Anterior view – schema only IVC shown

The veins have equivalents to the arterial brs with some exceptions. The inf. mesenteric vein draining to the splenic vein. The major veins drain to the portal vessels of the liver before emptying into the IVC. The azygos system also drains many of the GIT veins, particularly those of the oesophagus.

1-2 are hepatic vessels – Visceral vessels

1 middle hepatic v

2L left hepatic v – drains the L lobe of the liver

2R right hepatic v – large vein -drains the large R lobe of the liver

3 inferior phrenic v L = left / R = right

4 adrenal v L = left / R = right

5 renal v L = left / R = right

6 gonadal v L = left / R = right

7 common iliac v L = left / R = right

8 external iliac v

9 internal iliac v

10 median sacral v

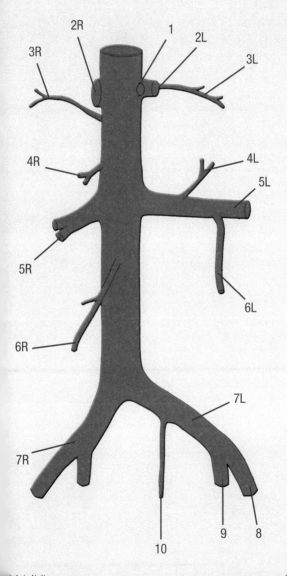

GIT overview – Blood Supply
Portal – Systemic anastomoses in the venous drainage

Schematic

Where the portal and systemic circulations meet there may be a pressure differential particularly in disease states and varicosities or distensions of the portal veins may occur, which if they rupture can lead to serious haemorrhages.

Clinically these may present as haemorrhoids & oesophageal varicosities.

1   azygos v
2   oesophageal v draining to azygos v
3   oesophageal v draining to L gastric v
4   stomach + oesophagus
5   portal / systemic aa = 3 + 2
site of oesophageal varicosities
6   splenic v
7   inf. mesenteric v
8   superior mesenteric v
9   venous drainage of LI and lower GIT
10 superior rectal vein -draining to inf mesenteric
11 inferior rectal – draining to int. iliac veins
12 portal / systemic aa = 10 + 11
site of haemorrhoids
13 anus
14 epigastric veins superior + inferior
15 paraumbilical v
16 portal / systemic aa = 14 + 15
site of "caput medusa" - ring vessels on the abdominal wall
17 liver
18 IVC

See also oesophagus and rectum

　　　　　　　　　　　　　　　　© A. L. Ne

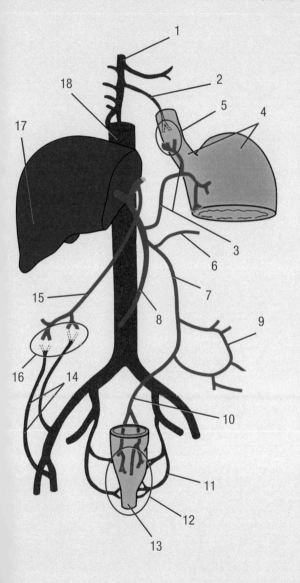

Wall of the GIT – Stomach

Schematic

Description: Throughout the GIT there are 4 layers with regional specializations.

A The Mucosa = the lining epithelium + the BM + the loose CT AKA Lamina propria (LP) composed of BVs, Lymphoid tissue (GALT), and Ns

B The Submucosa = LP lying deep to the mucosa and with similar components

C The Muscularis Externus = an inner circular layer of smooth muscle + an outer longitudinal layer containing an internal neural plexus – the myenteric plexus

D The Adventitia = Serosa = the CT surrounding the tube which supports the vascular and neural components

1 mucus lining of the stomach – very thick to protect the wall against the acid secretions

2 epithelial lining – single layer – shed regularly - protects against acid erosion

3 gastric glands – where HCL is produced – note as separate ions which combine in the lumen

4 muscularis mucosa – thin smooth muscle layer inner circular and outer longitudinal – increases the mobility of the mucosa

5 lymphoid tissue present in the mucosa & submucosa

6 circular layer of smooth muscle – with CT strands throughout

7 longitudinal spiral fibres of smooth muscle

8 serosa

9 visceral epithelium

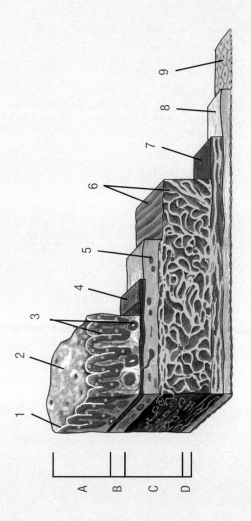

© A. L. Neill

Wall of the GIT – Small Intestine

Schematic

Description: Throughout the GIT there are 4 layers with regional specializations.

A The Mucosa = the lining epithelium + the BM + the loose CT AKA Lamina propria (LP) composed of BVs, Lymphoid tissue (GALT), and Ns

B The Submucosa = LP lying deep to the mucosa and with similar components

C The Muscularis Externus = an inner circular layer of smooth muscle + an outer longitudinal layer containing an internal neural plexus – the myenteric plexus

D The Adventitia = Serosa = the CT surrounding the tube which supports the vascular and neural components -

1 mucus coating of the small intestine – sticky to attract substances to the surface for absorption

2 epithelial lining – simple columnar cells with microvilli and glyocproteins on the surface, 1^0 function absorption + goblet cells

3 base of villi – site of cellular mitosis and migration to the villous tip – mucosal layer is very thick and vascular particularly at the jejunal - proximal end

4 muscularis mucosa – thin smooth muscle layer inner circular and outer longitudinal – increases the mobility of the mucosa

5 lymphoid nodules = Peyer's patches – very active immunologically may extend into the submucosa – protective against bacterial infiltration

6 circular layer of smooth muscle – with CT strands throughout

7 longitudinal fibres of smooth muscle – note these layers are very defined in the SI

8 serosa

9 visceral epithelium

10 central lymphatic vessel in the villous = lacteal and extensive lymphatic network

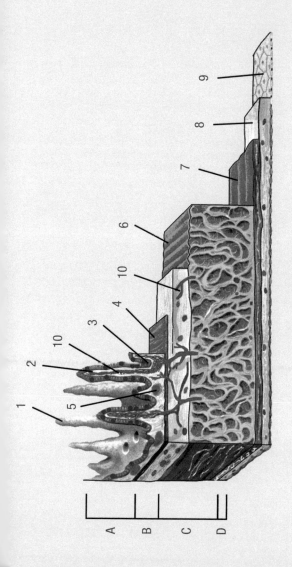

Wall of the GIT – Large Intestine

Schematic

Description: Throughout the GIT there are 4 layers with regional specializations.

A The Mucosa = the lining epithelium + the BM + the loose CT AKA Lamina propria (LP) composed of BVS, Lymphoid tissue (GALT), and Ns

B The Submucosa = LP lying deep to the mucosa and with similar components

C The Muscularis Externus = an inner circular layer of smooth muscle + an outer longitudinal layer containing an internal neural plexus – the myenteric plexus

D The Adventitia = Serosa = the CT surrounding the tube which supports the vascular and neural components -

1 mucus lining of the intestine – thick to lubricate the faecal material

2 epithelial lining – simple columnar Goblet cells

3 intestinal glands – mainly mucous cells limited absorptive function

4 muscularis mucosa – thin smooth muscle layer inner circular and outer longitudinal – increases the mobility of the mucosa

5 lymphoid nodules and tissue

6 circular layer of smooth muscle – with CT strands throughout

7 longitudinal fibres of smooth muscle –discontinuous layer limited to 3 bands of tissue - Taeniae libera

8 serosa

9 visceral peritoneal lining

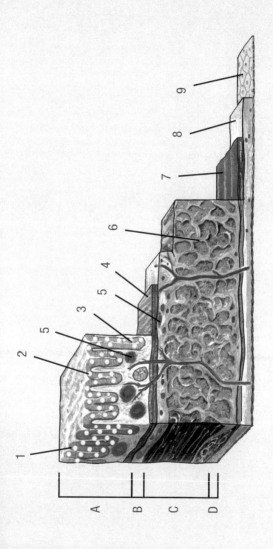

Face – muscles of expression and lip and cheek movement

Anterior – major muscles of the face

1. Frontalis muscle belly

2. Temporalis

3. muscles of the nose
   c = Compressor naris
   d = Dilator naris
   s = Depressor septi nasi

4. 4L Levator anguli oris

   4D Depressor anguli oris

5. Masseter

6. Buccinator

7. Risorius

8. Orbicularis oris

9. Depressor labii inferioris

10. Mentalis

11. Platysma – on both the lower face & neck

12. split in the Platysma may widen with age leading to softening and heaviness of the jawline sagging of the chin skin

13. Zygomaticus M = Major, m = minor

14. Levator labii superioris
    n = Levator labii superioris alaeque nasi

15. Orbicularis oculi

16. Depressor supercili

17. Corrugator

18. Procerus

19. Epicranius = Frontalis + Galea aponeurosis + Occipitalis (not seen)

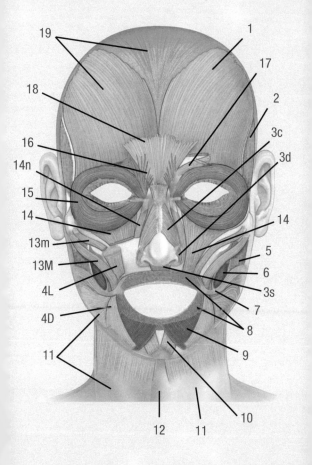

Muscles of the Face – Expression

Anterolateral view

Description: These muscles are often involved in cosmetic surgery and their function may be compromised by incisions at the level of the deep fascia.

1 Buccinator

2 Corrugator supercili

3 Depressor anguli Oris

4 Depressor labii inferioris, (overlying incisivus inf.)

5 Depressor septi

6 Frontalis (of occipitofrontalis)

7 Levator anguli oris (caninus),

8 Levator labii superioris

9 Levator labii superioris alaeque nasi
   (overlying Incisivus sup.)

10 Mentalis

11 Nasalis (compressor & dilator)

12 Orbicularis oculi

13 Orbicularis oris

14 Platysma

15 Procerus

16 Risorius

17 Zygomaticus major

18 Zygomaticus minor

NS facial N (CN VII) - supplies most of the muscles of the face
BS facial

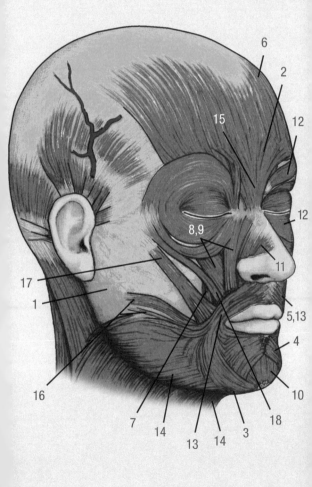

Mastication *Coronal section posterior view*

Primary movers of the Mandible + chewing and initiation of swallowing.

Muscles of mastication are all attached to the Mandible (Jaw bone) and are part of the Splanchnocranium. Those initiating swallowing move the food to the back of the throat & then into the oropharynx.

19 Masseter (F = Fascia)

20 Pterygoids Lateral (deep to Masseter)

21 Pterygoids Medial (deep to Buccinator)

22 Temporalis

NS trigeminal N –mandibular branch (CN V$_3$)
BS trigeminal and facial branches

Articulation & Swallowing

Primarily involved in speech and initiation of swallowing. They are often involved in "Stroke" patients affecting both speech and eating. *Not all demonstrated here.

31 Genioglossus

32 Geniohyoid

33 Styloglossus*

34 Hypoglossus

35 Stylohyoid*

36 Thyrohyoid*

37 Sternohyoid*

38 Sternothyroid*

39 Mylohyoid

40 Digastric*

NS hypoglossal (CN XII) and C1-3 of ansa cervicalis
BS facial a & branches

50 Mandibular sling = insertion raphe

51 Mandibular condyle

52 Interarticular disc of the TMJ

53 Sphenoid

See Muscles of the Hyoid.

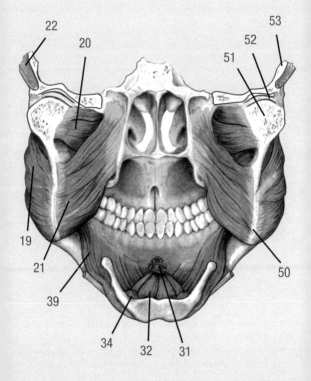

Muscles of Mastication – Chewing Masseter, Temporalis

Lateral view – Temporalis cut to show the medial Pterygoid

Description: Biting involves 2 muscles – Masseter & Temporalis and the teeth – Chewing involves 3 others the Buccinator & the Pterygoids and the Tongue.

There is a close association b/n these structures & the salivary glands.

1 Temporalis – attached to the conoid process of the Mandible (not shown)

2 Zygoma

3 Maxilla

4 Buccinator

5 incisor tooth

6 Masseter m

7 Sublingual salivary gland – smallest gland

8 Parotid gland - largest – most serous gland

9 Submandibular gland

10 angle of the jaw

11 medial pterygoid m

12 EAM

13 TMJ

for more details of the bones & muscles see the A to Z of the Head & Neck muscles & bones (note some texts use the terms internal and external Pterygoids to represent the medial and lateral respectively)

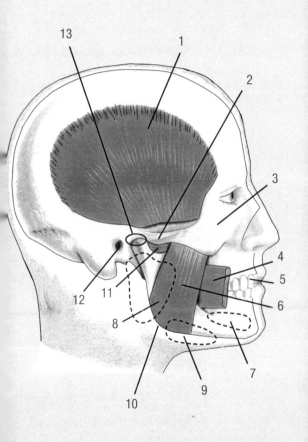

Muscles of the Hyoid bone & Thyroid cartilage (Larynx)

The Hyoid bone and the Larynx hang b/n the SUPRA-HYOID and INFRAHYOID muscles

They move with swallowing, breathing and speech

SWALLOWING cannot commence w/o the Mandible being fixed

It cannot continue w/o the Sternum and Clavicle being fixed to allow for the Hyoid to be depressed

Arrows show the directions of the muscles

These muscles determine the chin line and are involved in cosmetic surgery – Several muscles rely on tendinous slings and have two bellies to function.

Elevator Muscles

1 Palatoglossus

2 Stylopharyngeus

3 Thyrohyoid

4 Pharyngeal constrictors

5 Stylohyoid

6 Geniohyoid

7 Digastric m this muscle has 2 bellies ant & post

8 Mylohyoid

Depressor Muscles

9 Sternohyoid

10 Omohyoid

11 Sternothyroid

3 Thyrohyoid (both functions)

NS ansa cervicalis C1-3
BS facial and thyroid vessels

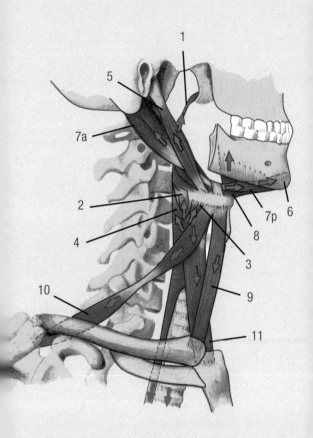

© A. L. Neill

Muscles of the Pharynx

Lateral

Description: The space b/n the mouth and oesophagus – a modified muscular tube directing the food bolus to the GIT.

Lifting the Pharynx closes the auditory tube and nasopharynx (10,11) food moves to the back of the throat – swallowing begins coordinated by the constrictors (1). It is supported by ligs (3,12) & muscles (2).

NS facial, maxillary
BS CN X – vagus, branches of ansa cervicalis (C1-3)

1 Pharyngeal constrictors m
   i = inferior
   m = middle
   s = superior
2 Stylopharyngeus m
3 Stylohyoid lig
4 Thyroid cartilage
5 Thyrohyoid membrane
6 Hyoid bone
7 Mylohyoid m
8 Mandible
9 Buccinator m
10 Palatopharyngeus m
11 Salpingopharyngeus m
12 Cricothyroid m
13 Oesophagus
14 Trachea

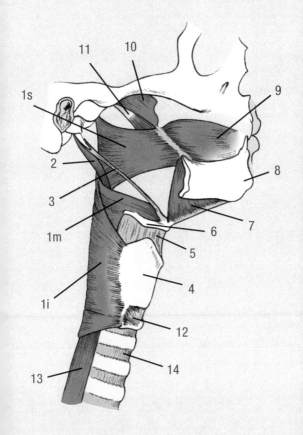

Muscles of the Tongue – overview

Coronal

Sagittal

Description: The tongue is a "bag of muscles" with a fixed pharyngeal root and free oral tip / apex. Muscles which move it from w/in are intrinsic and those which change its position from w/out are extrinsic.

Extrinsic

Genioglossus (4) - attaches to the Hyoid, Pharyngeal constrictors, Hypoglossus and intrinsic Lingualis muscles to protrude the tongue (poke out the tongue) depress the centre and raise the sides (make a tunnel with the tongue)

Hyoglossus (3) - attaches to the front and horns of the Hyoid, side of the tongue and intrinsic Lingualis muscles in order to depress the tongue (as in say AHHHHH…)

Palatoglossus (5) – attached to the palatine aponeurosis & blends with the lateral Linguali muscles

Styloglossus (2) - attaches to the styloid process, and blends with the Hypoglossus, Stylohyoid

Intrinsic

Linguali muscles (1)- superior, inferior, transverse and vertical

attach w/in the tongue to change its shape for speech, in mastication and swallowing

NS lingual, sublingual and hypoglossal (CN XII) Ns
BS lingual, sublingual and external carotid

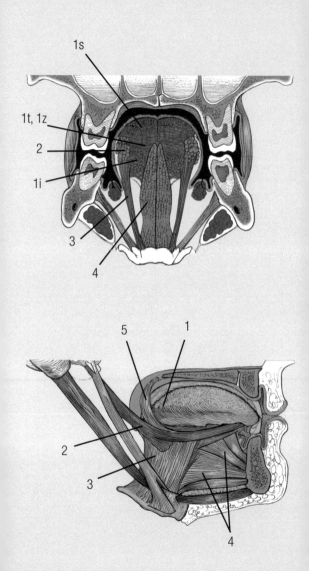

Swallowing – process

Schematic A initiation of swallowing
*   B completion of swallowing*

Description: Food bolus is moved to the back of the throat (ant. pharyngeal surface)

via the tongue (2) and mastication muscles -

The swallowing reflex is initiated

Pharyngeal muscles + Hyoid (3) – are raised and move forward

Soft Palate (9) is raised and closes off the Nasopharynx

Food bolus is moved onto the Vallecula of the Epiglottis (6)

Epiglottis is pushed posteriorly and closes the Trachea (4)

Food bolus passes into the Oesophagus (5)

Hyoid is lowered and Nasopharynx (10) opened

Epiglottis "bounces back" anteriorly and Trachea is opened

1 Oral cavity = mouth
2 Tongue
3 Hyoid bone
4 Tracheal passage
5 Oesophageal cavity
6 Epiglottis v = Vallecula
7 Oropharynx
8 Food bolus
9 Soft palate
10 Nasopharynx
11 Hard Palate
12 Nasal cavity
13 closure of the Nasopharynx
14 closure of the Tracheal passage

A

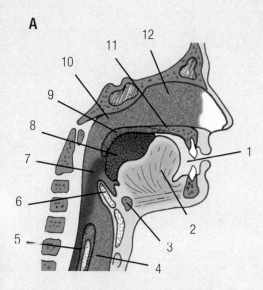

B

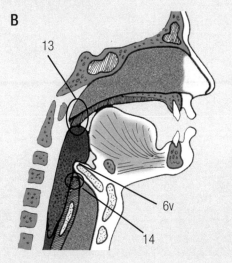

Salivation reflex (CN I, II, VII, IX higher emotional centres, sympathetic and parasympathetic fibres)

The thought, smell, sight or taste of food causing reflex secretion from the salivary glands

1 imput from higher centres - thinking of food

2 imput from seeing food Optic N = CN II - looking at food

3 imput from smelling food Olfactory N = CN I - smelling food

4a imput from tasting food Lingual N, Chorda Tympani (CN VII)

4b & Glossopharyngeal Ns (CN IX) - tasting food*

5 Solitary nucleus of Medulla = Nucleus Solitarius

6a Salivatory centres of the Facial

6b & Glossopharyngeal nuclei

7 Preganglionic sympathetic cells
(in the lateral horn of the SC) and fibres

8 Sympathetic chain

9 Postganglionic sympathetic fibres (↑ salivation)

10a Parasympathetic efferent fibres of CN IX and the Otic ganglion (↑ salivation)

10b Parasympathetic efferent fibres of CN VII and the Submandibular ganglion (↑ salivation)

11 Salivary gland

note trained reflexes of timing and signals such as aural input can also influence the afferent stimulus to salivate - also both parasympathetic and sympathetic fibres increase salivation

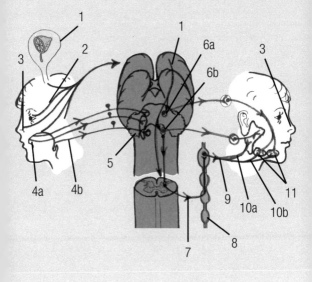

Swallowing reflex (CN IX, X, XII V$_3$)

a bolus of food or liquid - including saliva, placed at the back of the throat will cause the reflex initiation of swallowing

1. oropharynx
2. afferent fibres of Glossopharyngeal N (CN IX)
3. Solitary nucleus = Nucleus Solitarius
4. Nucleus Ambiguus (motor nucleus of CN IX X & XII)..
5. Vagus N (CN X)
6. Hypoglossal N (CN XII)
7. Preganglionic sympathetic cells (in the lateral horn of the SC) and fibres
8. Sympathetic chain
9. Postganglionic sympathetic fibres
10. interneuron connections stimulating peristalsis to the stomach
11. stomach

Gag reflex (CN X)

irritation of the oropharynx / larynx w/o swallowing imput will cause coughing and gaging and if severe vomiting

CN IX / X afferents will loop and efferent Ns will cause reflex reaction of coughing and muscle spasm

(Pharyngeal Constrictors)

diminished in 20% of people unless severely irritated - important to stop particles from going into the trachea

Jaw Jerk (CN V$_3$)

the mouth is opened slightly - strike the chin with a reflex hammer - jaw will close and then open rapidly -monosynaptic stretch reflex - (Masseter, Medial Pterygoid and Temporalis)

1. Temporalis
2. Masseter
3. Mandibular afferents (CN V$_3$)
4. Trigeminal ganglion
5. Proprioceptive nucleus
6. Motornucleus of Trigeminal N (CN V$_3$)
7. Efferents from Trigeminal N to muscles of mastication (CN V$_3$)

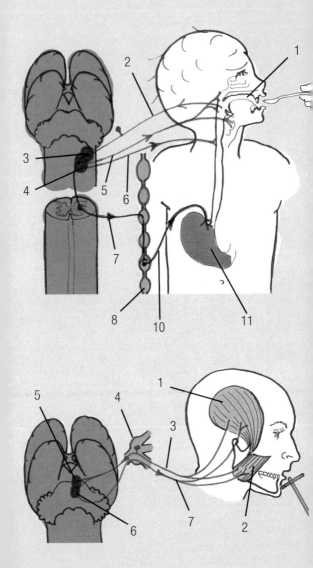

Defaecation – process

Schematic

Description: Faecal bolus is moved to the rectum
stimulating the autonomic = involuntary NS and a wave of peristalsis
the defaecation reflex
the bolus is moved the anal canal
the IAS relaxes and allows the bolus to exit unless overridden
unconsciously by UMN

1 Voluntary pathway – motor Ns from S 2,3,4 to EAS

2 Autonomic pathway – reflex arc to IAS

3 Sensory fibres detecting mass in the rectum

4 Sigmoid colon

5 Rectum

6 IAS

7 EAS

8 anal canal

9 motor fibres to EAS

10 motor fibres to IAS

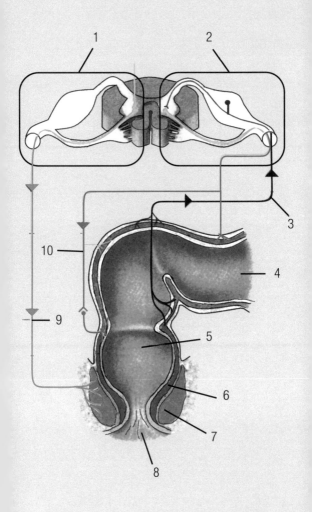

Neural pathways – the Parasympathetic control of the GIT via the Vagus (CN X)

Schematic – input of the Vagus into the functions of the GIT, tongue, oesophagus and upper GIT

Description: The GIT has its own internal NS but this can be modified by the ANS mainly the Vagus N – parasympathetic component which has a general stimulatory effect on the digestion process. It increases gallbladder, pancreatic and salivary secretions, gastric motility, and direct BF to the gut area.

1 input from the CC

2 pons

3 solitary tract and nucleus

4 nucleus ambiguous

5 dorsal vagal nucleus

6 SC

7g phrenic N nucleus

7n phrenic N

8 diaphragn

9 stomach

10n CN X = Vagus N

10p oesophageal plexus

11 physiological (smooth muscle) sphincter

12 crura of the diaphragm

13 oesophagus

14 tongue

15 pharynx

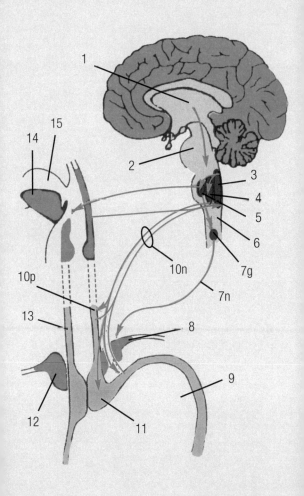

The Vagus N = CN X & the GIT

Schematic – input of the Vagus into the functions of the DT

Description: The GIT has its own internal NS but this can be modified by the ANS mainly the Vagus N – parasympathetic component which has a general stimulatory effect on the digestion process. It increases GB, pancreatic & salivary secretions, gastric & SI motility, and direct BF to the gut area.

1 Meningeal br of the Vagus N

2 Auricular br of the Vagus N

3 Glossopharyngeal N

4 Salpingopharyngeus m

5 Levator veli palatini m

6 Palatoglossus m

7 Palatopharyngeus m

8 Pharyngeal constrictors m

9 internal br of the Vagus

10 external br of the Vagus

11 Oblique & Transverse Arytenoid m

12 Thyroarytenoid m

13 Lat. Cricoarytenoid m

14 Post. Cricoarytenoid m

15 Recurrent Laryngeal N

16 Cardiac plexus N

17 Vagal trunks a = ant. p = post.

18 Stomach

19 Coeliac plexus N

20 SI

21 Ascending colon

22 Kidney, Adrenal gland, Spleen

23 Pancreas

24 Liver + GB

25 Thoracic aorta

26 Pulmonary plexus N

27 Oesophagus

28 Common carotid a

29 Cervical br of Vagus N i = inf. s = superior

30 Superior laryngeal N

31 Vagus N

32 Pharyngeal br of the Vagus N

33 Vagal ganglia I = Inf s = superior

34 Accessory N – Spinal and cranial roots

35 Jugular foramen

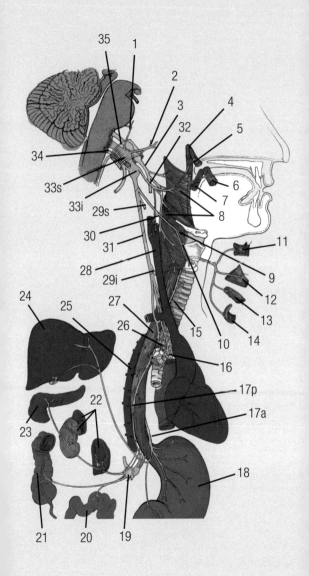

Neural pathways – Smell

Schematic - Inferior view - looking up from below to the base of the brain

Superior view - looking down into the ACF – cranial exit

Magnified Sagittal view - through Olfactory bulb and rootlets into and through the nasal mucosa

Description: The special sensation of smelling is provided by the Olfactory N – CN 1 - which functions as a brain extension.

Without an active sense of smell, taste is compromised and may be perceived differently. It was neurons from this N which were first used as stem cells.

1 Olfactory bulb
2 Olfactory tract
3 Mitral cell
4 Fibrous processes of receptor cells
5 Ethmoid bone with "olfactory holes" – in the Cribiform plate to allow passage of olfactory receptor N cell axons
6 Mucosa & CT for BVs and support to the Ns
7 Receptor cells
8 Basal cells of the nasal epithelium
9 Columnar epithelial cells
8 + 9 = nasal epithclium
10 Glycocalyx on apical surface of the epithelial cells - sticky
11 Mucous secreted from the nasal glands
12 Nasal glands
13 Long microvilli and knob – specialized endings of the receptor cells

See also nose and nasal cavity

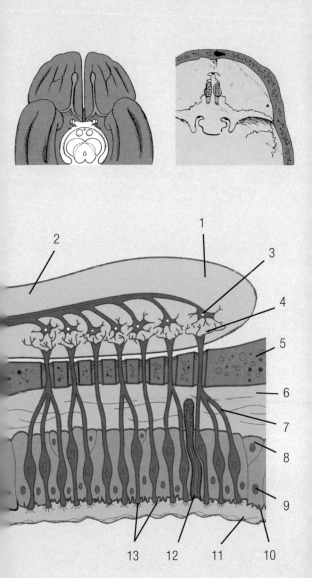

Neural pathways – Smell

Sagittal section – through the middle of the Head

Coronal section – through the facial sinuses

The Olfactory N – pure special sensory SMELL – functions as a brain extension.

Origin the olfactory bulb (3)

Course rootlets from receptor cells (4) in the nasal lining of the nasal cavity (6) at the superior concha (1) pass up through the Cribiform plate (2) of the Ethmoid bone synapse in the bulb (3) and sensory information then moves to the main brain tissue via the olfactory tracts (1) projecting to the olfactory areas of the CC via the Stria (7, 8) see Rhiencephalon.

Cranial Exit cribiform plate (2)

Branches none

Lesions amnosia inability to smell (and often taste is affected)

Aetiology injury to the ACF (20)

1   Olfactory tract

2   Cribiform plate (sieve)

3   Olfactory bulb

4   Olfactory N processes

5   Middle & inferior conchae

6   Nasal cavity

7   Medial stria

8   Lateral stria

9   Falx cerebri

10 ACF

11 Superior nasal concha

12 Sinus cavities – Sphenoid sinus

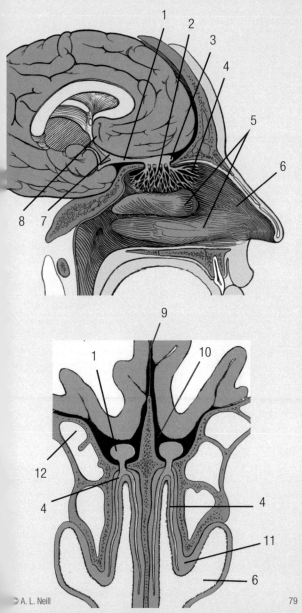

Tongue – Taste – Nerve Supply

Tongue macroscopic view of the dorsal surface
Taste bud histological section through the surface

The special sensation of Taste is supplied by 3 CNs on the ispilateral side with overlap b/n these Ns. Within these areas supplied are subareas which recognize specific taste types. However there is considerable variation and overlap of these areas.

The taste is detected via "taste buds" inserted into the stratified squamous epithelium of the tongue.

1　Taste pore

2　Microvilli

3　Supporting cells = sustenacular cells

4　Basal cell

5　Sensory N

6　Sensory N fibres into the cells

7　Sensory hair on cell surface

Areas on the tongue detect certain tastes more sensitively they do not reflect the innervation

A　SWEET area

B　SOUR area

C　SALTY area

D　BITTER area

CN VII　area innervated by the Chorda tympani - ant. tip of tongue

CN IX　area innervated by the Hypoglossal N - ant. 2/3 of tongue

CN X　area innervated by the Vagus N post. - 1/3 of tongue

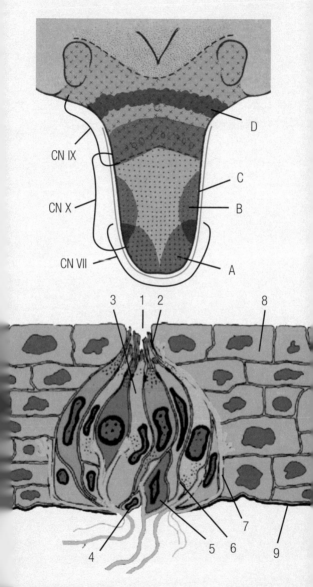

CN IX

CN X

CN VII

D

C

B

A

3 1 2

8

4 5 6 7 9

© A. L. Neill

Tongue – Taste – Nerve Supply

Afferent pathways

The special sensation of Taste is supplied by 3 CNs on the ispilateral side with overlap b/n these Ns.

Other sensory feedback such as pressure and pain is supplied by the Mandibular N (CN V_3), on the contralateral side.

1	ventroposteriomedical nuc of the Thalamus = arcuate and accessory arcuate nuclei of the Thalamus
2	solitariothalamic tract in the medical leminiscus
3	Brainstem
4	Fourth ventricle
5g	Trigeminal ganglion
5n	Spinal nucleus of CN V
5s	Sensory fibres of the Mandibular N
7g	Geniculate ganglion
7n	Sensory nucleus of Nervus intermedius = upper portion of Nucleus solitarius
7ss	Chorda Tympani fibres = special sense Taste fibres
8	Vallate papillae
9g	inf petrosal ganglion of CN IX
9s	Gustatory nucleus (part of the Nucleus Solitarius – solitary tract)
9ss	Special sensory fibres of CN IX - taste
10g	nodose ganglion of CN X = inferior vagal ganglion
10s	Solitary nucleus = Solitary tract = Solitary fasciculus
10ss	Special sensory fibres of CN X - taste
38	Brodmann area for normal tongue sensation = uncus
40,43	Brodmann areas for TASTE = Opercular Insular region in the cerebral cortex

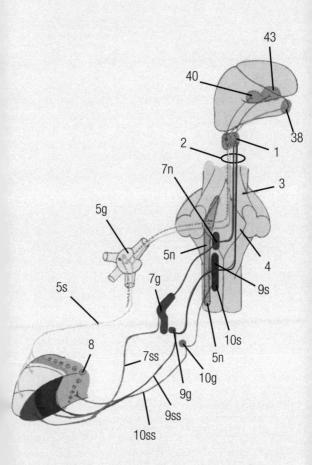

Tongue – surface

Superior – Schematic

Description: The tongue is "a bag of highly mobile skeletal muscle" - one of the strongest muscles in the body, covered with a tough stratified epithelium in which specialized epithelial structures are inserted - lined with taste buds, along with mucus and salivary glands.

1 Papillae of the tongue

2 Epithelial surface

3 Basement membrane

4 Mucus + Salivary glands

5 Skeletal muscle

Papillae of the tongue lined with Taste buds – morphology of papillae

A circumvallate

B conical

C filiform

D fungiform

E lenticular

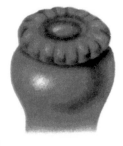
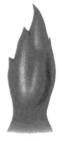
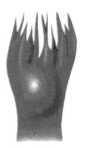

A   **B**   **C**

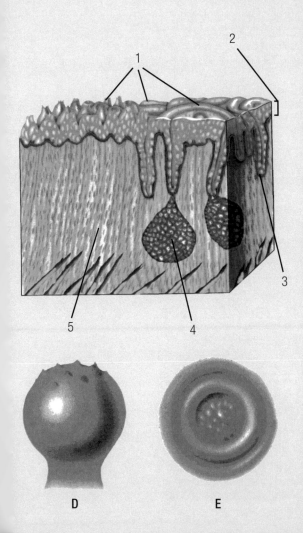

D

E

The Digestive Tract — Components

Bone, Glandular, Immune, Muscular (skeletal ±
smooth), Nervous, Other

Abdominal recesses *see Abdominal wall - posterior*

Abdominal wall

Abdominal wall — posterior

Adenoids = Pharyngeal tonsil *see Mouth & Throat overviews*

Anal Canal *see Anus*

Anal Sphincters

Anus *see also Rectum*

Appendices epiploiciae *see Appendix Colon*

Appendix AKA Vermiform Appendix *see also Colon*

Apron *see Omentum*

Ascending colon = R Colon *see Colon, Ileocaecal, junction*

Auerbach's plexus = myenteric plexus *see Oesophagus*

Bile duct *see also Gallbladder, Pancreas, Pancreatic duct*

Bite *see Teeth*

Brünner's glands *see Duodenum*

Buccinator *see muscles of mastication*

Caecum AKA Cecum *see Appendix, Ileocaecal junction Colon*

Coeliac trunk *see also Stomach*

Colon

Constrictors = Pharyngeal constrictors *see Pharynx, Throat*

Cystic Duct *see Gall Bladder*

Descending colon = L colon *see Colon*

Digastricus *see muscles of swallowing (overviews)*

Diverticulum

Duodenal flexure *see Duodenum*

Duodenum *see also Jejunum, Pancreas, Stomach*

Epiglottis *see Swallowing, Throat (overviews), Oesophagus, Pharynx*

Esophagus AKA Oesophagus

Facial N *see Nerves - Special functions & senses of the DT*

Flexures — Duodenal *see Duodenum Hepatic & Splenic see Colon*

Gall Bladder *see also, Bile duct, Coeliac trunk, Cystic duct, Liver*

Gallstones *see Gall Bladder*

Gastric Mucosa *see GIT overview micro-anatomy*

Gastro-intestinal tract = GIT *see DT overview, Colon*

Gastro-oesophageal junction *see Hiatus hernia*

Genioglossus

Geniohyoid

Glossopharyngeal N *see Nerves - Special functions & senses of the DT*

Greater omentum *see Omentum*

Greater sac *see Omental bursa*

Haemorrhoids *see Anus, Rectum*

Haustra = Haustrations *see Colon*

Hepatic artery – variations of... *see Gall Bladder*

Hepatic duct *see Gall bladder, Bile duct, Liver*

Hepatic flexure *see Colon*

Hiatus Hernia

Hyoid *see overviews - floor of the mouth, muscles of swallowing, Tongue*

Hypoglossal N *see Nerves - Special functions & senses of the DT*

Hypoglossus *see Tongue*

Ileocaecal junction

Ileocaecal valve *see Ileocaecal junction, Colon*

Ileum *see Small Intestine*

Inferior Lingualis *see Tongue*

Inferior mesenteric art / vein *see Colon*

Inferior Pharyngeal Constrictor *see Pharynx, Throat*

Intestine *see DT overview, GIT overview*

Islets of Langerhans *see Pancreas*

JAW = Mandible +Maxilla + Teeth *see Mouth overview*

Jejunum *see Duodenum, Small Intestine*

Lacteals *see SI, Villi*

Large intestine = Colon + Anus & Rectum *see Colon*

Lateral Pterygoid *see muscle groups and their functions in the DT*

Lesser omentum *see Omentum Omental Bursa*

Lesser sac *see Omental bursa*

Levator Anguli Oris (Caninus) *see Muscles of facial expression overviews*

Levator Ani *see Anus, Rectum*

Ligament of Treitz = Suspensory muscle of the Duodenum *see Duodenum*

Linguali muscles = Intrinsic muscles of the Tongue *see Tongue overview*

Lips *see also Mouth overview*

Liver

Liver lobules *see Liver*

Lymph nodules = Lymph follicles
see Abdominal wall - posterior, GIT structure overview

Lymphoid tissue of the Gut = GALT
see SI, Mouth and Throat overviews

Mandible = JAW = lower jaw *see Mouth overview*

Mandibular N *see Mouth overview - Jaw NS*

Masseter *see Muscles of Mastication*

Maxilla = upper jaw *see Mouth overview*

Maxillary artery *see mouth overview - Jaw BS*

Maxillary N *see Nerves - Special functions & senses of the DT mastication.*

Medial Pterygoid *see muscle groups and their functions in the DT*

Meissner's plexus = submucosal plexus *see Oesophagus*

Mesentery

Mesentery attachments – *see Abdominal wall - posterior*

Modiolus *see Mouth overview*

MOUTH = oral cavity *see Mouth overview*

Mucous glands = mucus producing glands *see Salivary glands*

Muscularis Uvulae = Uvulae Muscularis, *see Mouth overview*

Myenteric plexus = Auerbach's plexus *see Oesophagus*

Mylohyoid *see Mouth overview*

Nasopharynx *see Nose, Pharynx, Throat overview*

NOSE = nasal cavity and surrounding structures
see also special senses in overview – Smell

Oesophagus (AKA Esophagus) *see also Hiatus hernia, Stomach*

Omental bursa

Omentum

Oral Cavity = MOUTH *see Mouth overview*

Orbicularis Oris *see Lips, Mouth overview*

Orophaynx *see Pharynx, Throat*

Palate *see Mouth overview*

Palatoglossus *see Mouth overview*

Palatopharyngeus *see Mouth overview*

Pancreas *see also Bile duct, Duodenum*

Pancreatic duct variations *see Bile duct, Duodenum, Pancreas*

Parotid gland *see also Salivary glands*

Peritoneum = Peritoneal cavity *see also Abdominal wall - posterior*

Peyer's Patches = Lymphoid nodules *see GIT micro-anatomy overviews*

Pharyngeal Constrictors *see Pharynx, Throat*

Pharynx *see also Throat overview*

Plicae circularis *see Duodenum*

Polyp *see Colon*

Portal circulation *see GIT BS overview, Liver*

Posterior abdominal wall *see Abdominal wall - posterior*

Pterygoids *see muscle groups and their functions in the DT overviews*

Pyloris *see Stomach*

Rectum *see also Anus*

Salivary glands *see also Mouth overview, Parotid, Sublingual*

Submandibular glands

Salpingopharyngeus *see Pharynx, Throat overviews*

Serous glands *see Salivary glands*

Sigmoid colon *see Anus, Colon, LI, Rectum*

Sinusoids *see Liver*

Small Intestine = SI *see also Duodenum, GIT overviews, Villi*

Sphincter Ani = Anal Sphincters

Sphincter of Oddi *see Duodenum*

Splenic Flexure *see Colon*

Sternohyoid *see Muscles of swallowing*

Sternothyroid *see Muscles of swallowing*

Stomach *see also Oesophagus, Portal anastomoses*

Styloglossus *see Tongue muscle overview*

Stylohyoid *see Tongue muscle overview*

Stylopharyngeus *see Tongue muscle overview*

Sublingual salivary glands *see also Salivary glands*

Submandibular glands *see also Salivary glands*

Submucosal plexus = Meissner's plexus *see Oesophagus*

Superior Lingualis *see Tongue Muscle overview*

Superior mesenteric art/vein *see BS of the GIT overview, Colon, SI, Stomach*

Suspensory muscle of the Duodenum *see Duodenum*

Taeni Coli = Muscular coli *see Colon*

Taste buds see Special senses overviews, taste, Tongue

Teeth overview

Teeth / Tooth / types

THROAT = Pharynx + *see overviews*

Temporalis see muscles of mastication
Temporoparietalis *see muscles of mastication*
Temporomandibular joint = TMJ
Tensor Veli Palatini *see Swallowing, Mouth overview Pharynx*
Thyroepiglotticus *see Mouth, swallowing overviews, Pharynx*
Thyrohyoid *see Mouth, swallowing overviews, Pharynx*
Tongue *see also Nerves & special functions of the DT*
Tonsils *see Mouth and Throat overviews*
Transverse Colon *see Colon, LI*
Transverse Linguali *see Tongue*
Trigeminal N *see mouth overview*
    Nerves - Special functions & senses of the DT

Vermiform Appendix = Appendix *see also Caecum, LI*
Vertical Lingualis *see Tongue*

Uvula *see Pharynx, Throat*

Villi *see also Small intestine*

Zygomaticus Major *see muscles of face and splanchnocranium*
Zygomaticus Minor *see muscles of face and splanchnocranium*

Notes...

A Abdominal Wall

B GIT projection

Anterior view of the abdomen showing the GIT projected.

1. xiphisternum
2. oesophagus - *enters the abdomen at T10, L of the midline*
3. spleen
4. fundus of the stomach - *stomach fills the epigastric region, varies in size partially covered by the ribcage*
5. costochondral border
6. pyloris antrum ⇨ to pyloric sphincter
7. duodenum - first part - *begins R of midline below transpyloric plane*
8. descending duodenum - second part
9. horizontal duodenum - third part
10. duodenojejenal flexure - *midline T12 subcostal plane*
11. terminal ileum - *in RIF*
12. appendix - *2/3 of line from ASIS to umbilicus*
13. caecum - *RIF closely assoc with appendix*
14. ascending colon - *retroperitoneal structure*
15. transverse colon - *attached to mesentery*
16. splenic flexure -
17. descending colon - *retroperitoneal structure*
18. sigmoid colon - *attached to mesentery*
19. iliac tubercle
20. ASIS

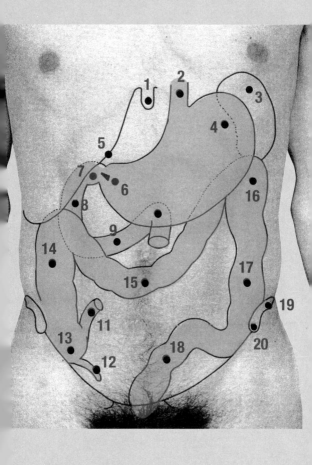

A Abdominal Wall

B Accessory Alimentary structures projection

C Anterior view of the abdomen showing the liver, pancreas & spleen.

1. **liver** - *fills the R hypochondrium, across to the epigastrium & above the CC to 4th ICS*
2. **gall bladder** - *MCL ∩ with the CC*
3. **spleen** - *post wall ribs 9-11*
4. **pancreas - body** - *stomach fills the epigastric region, varies in size partially covered by the ribcage*
5. **pancreas - tail** - *lodges in the hilum of the spleen*
6. **pancreas - head** - *lodges in the "C" of the duodenum*
7. **duodenum** -
8. **aortic bifurcation** - *ant. at the umbilicus - post. L4*
9. **IVC** - *midline to the R of the aorta - L5*
10. **external iliac artery** - *superior to inguinal lig at the MIP*
11. **femoral artery** - *inf to the inguinal lig*
12. **inguinal ligament**
13. **ASIS**
14. **iliac tubercle**

© A. L. Ne

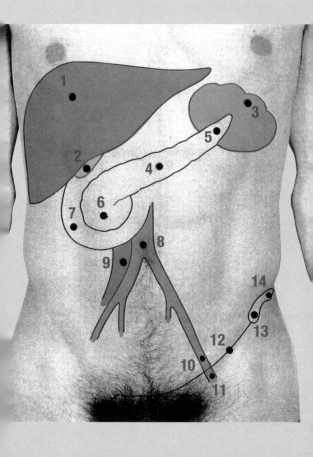

A Abdominal Wall

B Regions

C *Anterior view of the abdomen showing regions.*

D There are several ways to describe the regions of the Abdomen.

E This commonly used schema divides the abdomen into 9 regions, based upon anatomical landmarks - numbered

F Regions are coloured areas labelled with letters

G 1 Xiphisternum

H 2 midclavicular line (MCL) - *vertical line ½ way along the Clavicle*

I 3 transpyloric plane - *midway b/n Xiphisternum and umbilicus = L1 passes through pyloric sphincter and 1st part of the duodenum*

K 4 subcostal plane - *passes through L3*

L 5 transtubercular plane - *passes through L5*

M 6 Inguinal ligament

N 7 midinguinal point (MIP) - *intersection b/n MCL and inguinal lig*

O 8 anterior superior iliac spine = ASIS

P 9 iliac tubercle

10 7th rib - b= bone c = cartilage

Q 11 MCL ∩ 9th rib

R 12 CC - *lower border of the ribs from the Xiphisternum around*

S 13 umbilicus - varies with age & weight - T10 dermatome

T E = epigastrium - area b/n 3 & 12

U H = hypochondrium - area b/n MCL 3 & 4 L = left & R=right

V I = iliac region - area b/n MCL & 6 L = left & R = right

W L = lumbar region - area b/n MCL & 4 & 5 L= left & R = right

X P = pelvic area AKA suprapubic region - area below 5 above 6

Y

Z U = umbilical region - area b/n MCLs 4 & 5

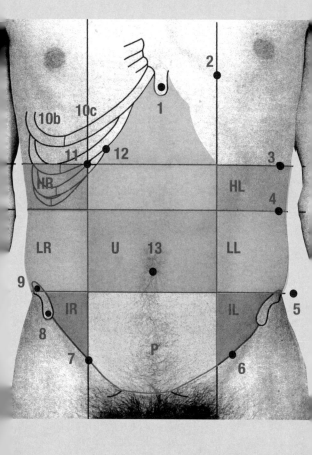

A Abdominal Wall

B Regions indicators of pain

Anterior view of the abdomen showing regions.

RH = HYPOCHONDRIUM Right lobe of liver Gallbladder Part of duodenum Hepatic flexure of colon Part of right kidney Suprarenal gland	E = EPIGASTRIUM Pyloric end of stomach Duodenum Pancreas Aorta Portion of liver	LH = HYPOCHONDRIUM Stomach Spleen Tail of pancreas Splenic flexure of colon Upper pole of left kidney Suprarenal gland
Gallstones Cholangitis Hepatitis Liver Abscess Cardiac & Lung pathology	Oesophagitis Pelvic Ulcer Perforated Ulcer Pancreatitis	Spleen Abscess Acute Splenomegaly Splenic rupture
RL = LUMBAR Ascending colon Lower half of right kidney Part of duodenum and jejunum	U = UMBILICAL REGION Omentum Mesentery Transverse colon Lower part of duodenum Jejunum and ileum	LL = LUMBAR Descending colon Lower half of left kidney Parts of jejunum and ileum
Ureteric Colic Pyelonephritis	Appendicitis (early) Mesenteric adenitis Meckel's diverticulitis Lymphomas	Ureteric Colic Pyelonephritis.
RI = ILIAC REGION Cecum Appendsix Lower end of ileum Right ureter Right ovary in female	P = PELVIC AREA AKA PUBIC REGION AKA HYPOGASTRIC REGION Ileum Bladder	LI = ILIAC REGION Sigmoid colon Left ureter Left ovary in female
Diverticulitis Ulcerative Colitis Constipation Ovarian Cyst Hernias	Testicular Torsion Urinary Retention Cystitis Placental Abruption	Diverticulitis Ulcerative Colitis Constipation Ovarian Cyst Hernias

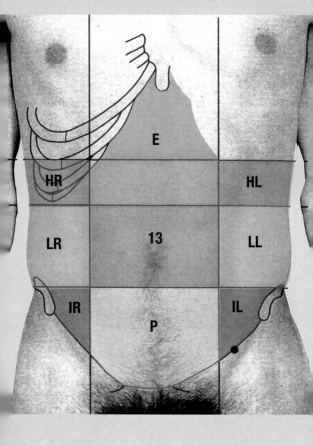

© A. L. Neill

A Abdominal Wall
B Incisions

C *Anterior view of the abdomen showing incision scars and*
D *their possible causes.*

E 1 **midline** - *approach for upper GIT tract*

2 **roof top** - *approach for adrenals and kidneys*
F
3 **renal** - *may also be more posterior*
G
4 **transverse** - *to approach the pyloric sphincter /*
H *gastroduodenal junction, partic in infants*

I 5 **laparoscopic point** - *for of the abdominal and*
J *pelvic organs*

K 6 **peritoneal catheter insertion**

L 7 **suprapubic** = *Pfannenstiel - approach for bladder*
uterus & adnexae Caesarean deliveries

M 8 **RIF** - *approach for appendix*

N 9 **subcostal** - *approach for GB and liver*

O 10 **paramedian** - *superior to inguinal lig at the*
mid inguinal pt
P
11 **access pt for liver biopsy** - *7th ICS axillary line*
Q

R

S

T

U

V

W

X

Y

Z

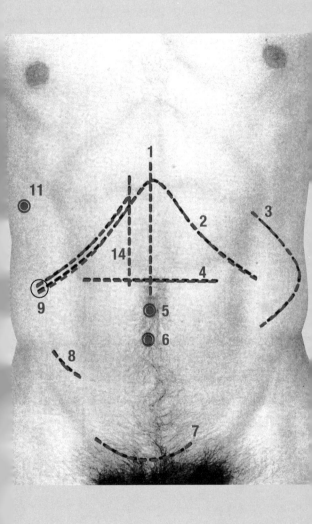

A Abdominal wall – Posterior
B Abdominal recesses

Schematic - Anterior view of the posterior abdominal wall, organs removed

Description: the posterior abdominal wall contains many organs some of which are fixed to its surface and immobile – retro – peritoneal and others attached via a mesentery from which it gains its BS, lymphatic drainage and NS – increased mobility. In order to access these structures and understand the way diseases or cancers spread, it is necessary understand their connections.

1 Subphrenic recesses L = left / R = right
2 Hepatogastric recess = Subhepatic recess
3 Omental bursa = Lesser sac
4 Duodenal recesses – inf / superior
5 Paracolic gutter L = left / R = right
6 Infracolic recesses L = left / R =right
7 Intersigmoiodal recess
8 Pelvic space
9 Retrocaecal recess
10 Ileocaecal recesses – inf./ superior
11 Hepatorenal recess = Morrison's recess
12 Coeliac trunk
13 Cardia = cardiac oesophagus into the stomach
14 Duodeno-jejenal flexure – opening
15 Sigmoid colon mesentery root
16 Rectum
17 Root of SI mesentery
18 Pyloris
19 Hepatoduodenal lig
20 Epiploic foramen

A B C D E F G H I J K L M N O P Q R S T U V W X Y Z

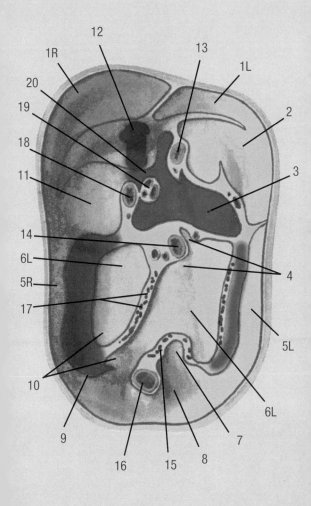

A Anal Sphincter – External =
B External Anal Sphincter = (EAS)

C *Schematic - looking onto the Sphincter from the side and up from below*

D **Definition:** the anus is the external opening of the DT, preceded by the anal canal and controlled by the anal sphincters a series of muscles which under voluntary and involuntary control determine the passage of faecal material.

G The EAS is under voluntary control (NS = S2, 3, 4) and consists of 3 parts. It lies inferior and is more superficial than Levator ani and the IAS.

It is normally contracted and relaxes to allow the passage of material.

1 Rectum

2 Puborectalis = anal sling

3 EAS - deep

4 EAS – superficial (inserting into the Peroneal body)

5 EAS – subcutaneous

6 Anus

7 Coccyx

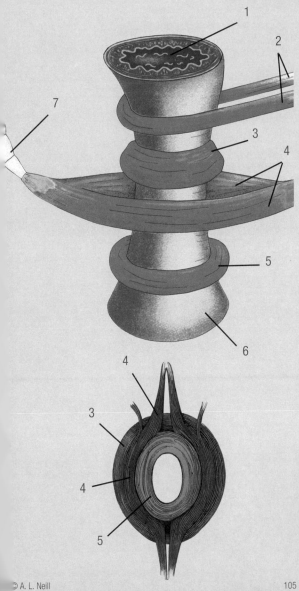

A Anus & Rectum

B *Anterolateral* - looking onto the DT cavities, wall opened to see
C the internal surfaces.

D **Definition:** the anus is the external opening of the DT, preceded by
the anal canal and controlled by the anal sphincters. The Rectum
E is superior - lying b/n the Sigmoid colon and anorectal line
(dentate line). Often the site of hemorrhoids - due to the meeting
F of the portal and systemic BS.

G 1 Sigmoid colon

H 2 Rectal valves i = inf / m = middle / s = superior

I 3 Muscular layers of the rectum – outer longitudinal /
inner circular – smooth muscle
J
4 Levator Ani m
K
5 EAS deep, superficial & subcut. parts
L
6 Fibrous septum
M
7 Corrugator cutis ani m
N
8 Anal glands – supplying lubrication in defecation
O
9 Anal columns – leading to the anal crypts on the
P Dentate line (note the serrated edge)
division b/n the anus and the rectum*
Q
10 Anal verge
R
11 Internal venous plexus in submucosa
S
12 IAS
T
13 Fat
U
14 Rectal fascia
V
15 Peritoneal fascia – reflected

16 Taeni coli of the Sigmoid colon – merging to form
W continuous layer in the Rectum

X * site of Hemorrhoids

Y

Z

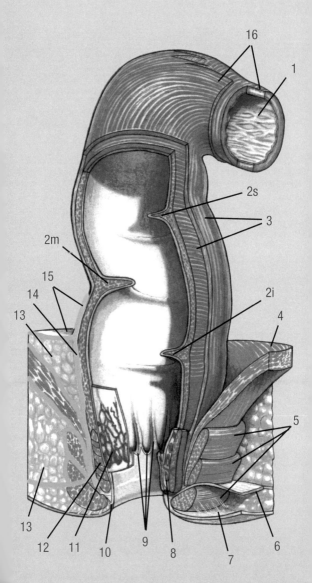

A Anus + Rectum in situ – fascial layers

B *Coronal*

C *Definition:* the anus and rectum are supported by the Levator Ani which borders the Ischiorectal fossa (= ischioanal fossa) the space filled with soft semi-liquid fatty material which allows for the shape changes of substances which pass through

1 Rectum
2 Pelvic fascia
3 Pelvic Diaphragmatic fascia inf /superior
4 Obturator internus
5 Ischio rectal fossa
6 EAS + IAS
7 Anus
8 Skin
9 Pudendal canal = Alcock's canal – containing Pudendal Artery, Nerve + Vein
10 Obturator fascia
11 Rectal fascia

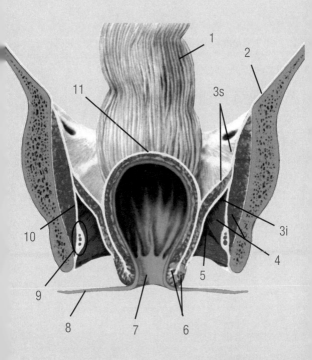

1

2

11

3s

10

9

8

7

6

3i

4

5

A Appendix = Vermiform Appendix – positions

Description: the appendix has its own mesentery and is very mobile. The pain of an inflamed appendix may present in several different locations. A ruptured appendix may spill its contents over several different organs of the peritoneum and this may result in serious consequences, such as the fibrosis of the ovary rendering it infertile.

1. Appendix (8-10cm)
   i = iliac
   p = pelvic
   r = retrocaecal – the commonest position – corresponding to McBirney's point

   2/3 of the line from the ASIS to the umbilicus

2. point of convergence of the taeniae coli – base of the appendix

3. inferior ileocaecal recess

4. mesoappendix = mesentery of the appendix

5. Ileum

6. branches of the appendicular artery

7. Caecum (5-7cm)

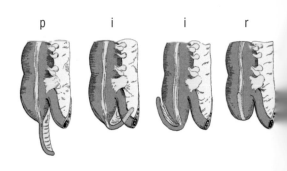

p   i   i   r

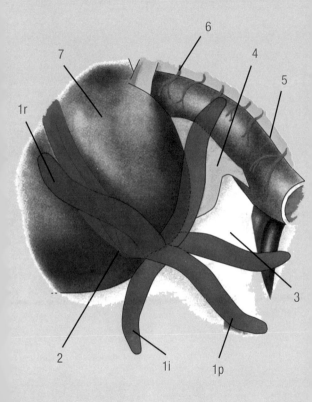

7

6

4

5

1r

2

1i

1p

3

A Appendix, Caecum Ileocaecal junction –
B Blood supply – Arterial

Anterior - wall cut away from caecum and mesentry removed from the BVs.

1. Mesentery (cut)
2. Ileum
3. straight arteries = arteriae rectae
4. arterial arcades
5. Appendicular a
6. Appendix v = appendix orifice
7. Ileocolic artery
   Brs –
   a = ant. caecal a
   c = colic a
   i = ileal a
   p = post. caecal a
8. Lymphatic follicules = Peyers' patches
9. Ascending colon

C
D
E
F
G
H
I
J
K
L
M
N
O
P
Q
R
S
T
U
V
W
X
Y
Z

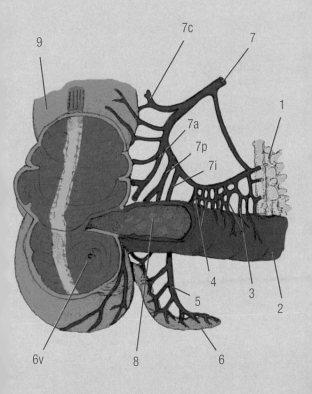

Coeliac Trunk = Celiac Trunk

Description: The first unbranched artery arising from the abdominal aorta, part of the GIT BS. It supplies the lower end of the oesophagus stomach and duodenum. The branches of the superior mesenteric and the coeliac art have a number of variations – the commonest are demonstrated here.

1 Fundus of the stomach

2 Diaphragm

3 Spleen

4 Gastroepiploic art. L = left , R = right

5 Aorta

6 Gastroduodenal a

7 Common hepatic a

8 Gastric art L = left, R = right

9 Coeliac trunk

10 IVC

11 R crus of the diaphragm

12 Oesophagus

13 Physiological sphincter of the diaphragm

14 Splenic a

15 Renal a – note this is not part of the GIT BS

16 Superior mesenteric a

17 Hepatic art. L = left, R = right branches

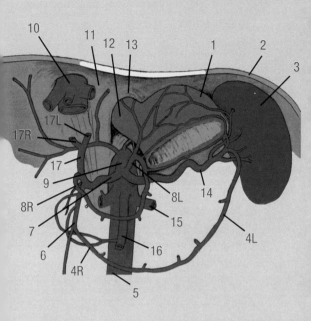

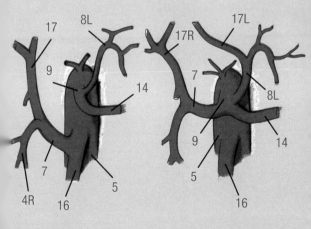

Colon – Large Intestine (LI)

Description: the Colon is a muscular tube up to 1.5 m long – divided into 4 parts which ring the abdominal cavity, fixed on the sides.

1 Ileum

2 Ileocaecal valve – site of Vitamin B12 & bile resorption

3 Vermiform appendix = Appendix

4 Caecum (5-7cm)

5 Lymphoid tissue and nodes in the mucosa

6 Ascending colon = R sided colon (12cm) fixed to the post abdominal wall – no mesentery

7 Hepatic flexure = R colic flexure inf to the liver

8 Transverse Colon = Horizontal Colon (45cm) has a mesentery which allows movement

9 Splenic flexure = L colic flexure – higher than the R - inf to the spleen

10 Appendices epiploiciae – small fat filled tags - increasing in size with increased fat storage

11 Taeniae Coli – one of 3 discontinuous layers of longitudinal muscles in the LI

12 Sigmoid colon = S – shaped colon (20-30cm) has a separate mesentery may store up to 2 kg of matter

13 Rectum – fixed

14 recto-anal junction

15 Levator Ani

16 Anus

17 internal semi-lunar valves

18 inner circular layer of smooth muscle

19 Mucosal surface

A
B
C
D
E
F
G
H
I
J
K
L
M
N
O
P
Q
R
S
T
U
V
W
X
Y
Z

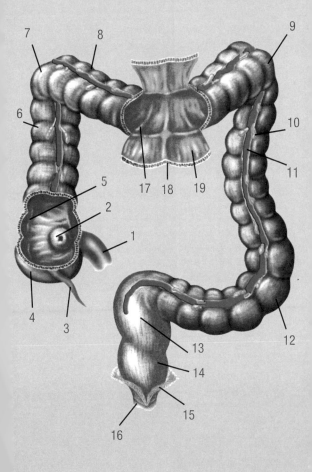

Colon – Blood Supply

Description: the arterial and venous BS of the Colon mirror each other. The superior mesenteric artery arises from the abdominal aorta and supplies the ascending and most of the TC; the inferior mesenteric artery supplies the rest. There are extensive overlaps and aas b/n the 2 vessels.

The superior mesenteric vein drains to the splenic vein; the inferior mesenteric vein to the portal vein.

1 Colon
   a = ascending
   d = descending
   t = transverse
   s = sigmoid

2 Rectum

3 Anus

4 Appendix

5 Superior mesenteric art /vein

6 R colic art/vein

7 Ileocolic art/ vein

8 Middle colic a / v

9 L colic a / v

10 Sigmoid a / v

11 Appendical branches of the ileocolic vessels

12 Abdominal aorta / Portal vein

13 Coelic trunk

14 Splenic v

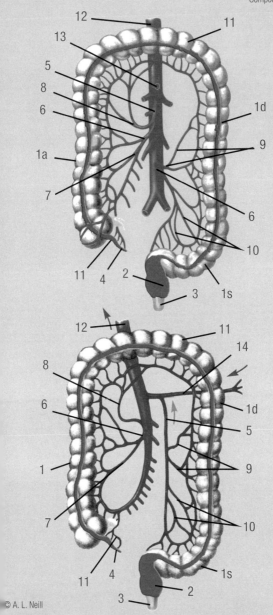

A
Colon – Large Intestine - lymphatics
B *Schematic - Anterior view of the peritoneum*
C *SI and organs removed showing LI and the lymphatics*

D **Description:** As with all structures along the GIT the intestines
have an extensive lymphatic drainage and rich vascularity. The BS
E of the SI enters via its supportive mesentery and the LNs lie along
the root of this mesentery. The LI is a fixed retroperitoneal
F structure for most of its length – its LNs flank its walls and follow
G its BS. The lymph drains to the thoracic duct.

H 1 thoracic duct
I 2 abdominal aorta
   3 coeliac nodes
J 4 epiploic LNs
K 5 paracolic LNs
L 6 posterior abdominal wall – outside the peritoneum + rib
M 7 inferior mesenteric LNs (+ art)
   8 L colic LNs
N 9 sigmoid LNs
O 10 pre-aortic LNs
P 11 superior rectal LNs
   12 bladder
Q 13 inguinal lig
R 14 appendicular LNs + mesentery
S 15 caecal LNs
   16 ileocolic LNs
T 17 R colic LNs
U 18 paracolic gutter
V 19 small intestine mesentery and BVs
   20 middle colic LNs
W 21 cisternae chyli
X 22 superior mesenteric LNs
Y 23 duojejunal junction

Z

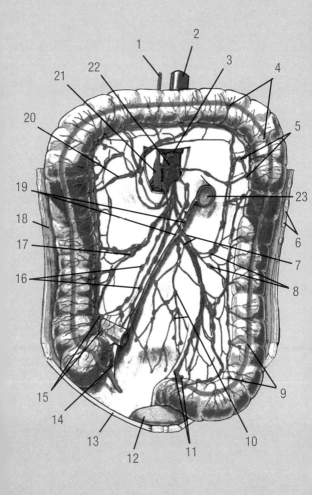

Duodenum – structure

Anterior – Stomach & TC removed

note the pancreas has been cut away to demonstrate the ducts

D *Definition:* the Duodenum is the 1st part of the SI = about 25cm
long and C – shaped. It is divided into 4 parts, retroperitoneal,
immovable, lies on the Psoas muscles, kidneys and adrenals and
encircles the pancreas. It receives secretions from the GB,
pancreas and its own highly alkaline mucous glands – Brünner's
glands. BS is from the coeliac trunk.

1 Duodenum
  a = 1st part = superior
  b = 2nd part = descending
  c = 3rd part = horizontal
  d = 4th part = ascending

2 Coeliac trunk

3 Adrenal gland

4 Kidney

5 Pancreas

6 Transverse mesocolon

7 Descending colon

8 Jejunum

9 Psoas major muscle

10 abdominal aorta

11 Superior mesenteric BVs

12 Pancreatic ducts – major + accessory + common

13 Transverse colon

14 Common bile duct

15 IVC

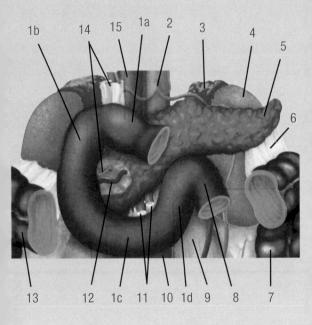

A # **Duodenum** – structure internal

B *Anterior – Stomach and TC removed*

C note the pancreas has been cut away to demonstrate the ducts
D and the wall opened to demonstrate the layers and structures.

E *Definition:* the Duodenum is the 1st part of the SI = about 25cm
long and divided into 4 parts. It is retroperitoneal and immovable. It
F receives secretions from the GB, pancreas and its own highly
alkaline mucous glands – Brünner's glands; specific to this section
G of the GIT. This mucus is important to reverse the acid chyme
H entering via the pyloric sphincter from the stomach.

I
- 1 Duodenum
   a = 1st part = superior   b = 2nd part = descending
J   c = 3rd part = horizontal   d = 4th part = ascending
K
- 2 Duodenal papilla – entrance of the pancreatic & bile
   ducts through a muscular sphincter
L
- 3 Kidney
M
- 4 Pancreas
N
- 5 Brünner's glands = duodenal glands – alkaline
O   mucous glands of the duodenum in the Submucosa
- 6 mucosa – permanent folds are present in parts
P   2,3,4
Q   plicae circulares (smooth mucosa in the 1st part)
- 7 thick smooth muscle layers – inner circular,
R   outer longitudinal
S
- 8 outer serosal covering
T
- 9 Abdominal aorta
U
- 10 Superior mesenteric BVs
V
- 11 Pancreatic ducts – major + accessory* + common
- 12 Transverse colon
W
- 13 Common bile duct
X

Y ** note the pancreatic duct may enter with the common bile duct in a
common opening or a separate opening. The accessory pancreatic duct
Z is only present in 30% of patients.*

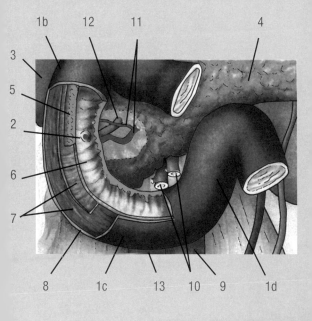

1b   12   11   4

3

5

2

6

7

8   1c   13   10   9   1d

A

Duodenum, Gall bladder, Pancreas &

B

Spleen – Blood supply Arterial

C

Stomach cut and removed – showing posterior structures

behind the stomach

D

most veins removed IVC remains

E

The stomach overlays the pancreas and duodenum, leaving a space

F

behind, bordered by the omenta. The head of the pancreas lies in

the curve of the duodenum. Branches of the coeliac trunk supply all

G

these structures and richly aa. The pancreas is retroperitoneal.

H

The duodenum has its own mesentery.

I

1	Spleen	16	Common hepatic a
2	L gastroepiploic a	17	Coeliac trunk
3	splenic vessels	18	GB
4	tail of the pancreas	18c	cystic a
4a	art. of the tail of the pancreas	19	branches of the Proper hepatic a
4d	dorsal art. of the pancreas	20	Gastric L&R a
4g	great pancreatic a	21	Inf. phrenic a
4h	head of the pancreas	22	Stomach – cut
4i	inf. pancreatic a		
5	splenic a		
6	body of the pancreas		
7	Jejunum		
8	middle colic a		
9	superior mesenteric v		
10	inf. pancreatoduodenal a		
11	R gastro-epiploic a		
12	Duodenum		
13	ant. sup. Pancreatoduodenal a		
14	Supraduodenal a		
15	Portal v		

J
K
L
M
N
O
P
Q
R
S
T
U
V
W
X
Y
Z

© A. L. Ne

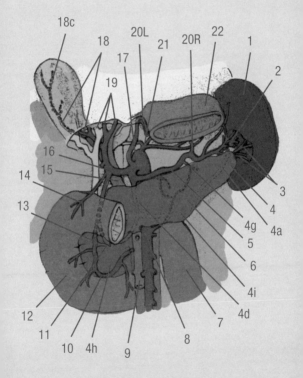

A # **Diverticulum**

B *Anterior*

C *Description:* a significant outpouching of the SI occurs in 2-4% of
D people Merkel's diverticulum and may be up to 7 cm long.
It generally occurs in the Ileum 10 cm from the ileocaecal valve.
E It may twist and mimic the symptoms of appendicitis – and may
contain ectopic gastric mucosa or pancreatic glandular tissue.
F

G 1 Ileum

H 2 SI mesentery

I 3 Diverticulm

J

K

L

M

N

O

P

Q

R

S

T

U

V

W

X

Y

Z

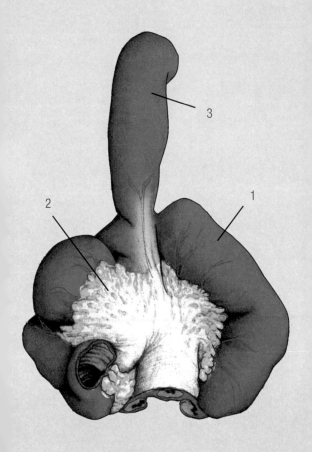

A

Gall Bladder and Ducts

B *Definition:* the gall bladder (GB) holds excess bile produced by the
C liver – releasing it into the duodenum when stimulated by fat. Bile
from the liver runs down the hepatic ducts (1, 2) until it reaches
D the duodenal papilla (8), w/o release it then travels back up to the
E GB where it is stored and concentrated. The bile and the
pancreatic secretions meet at the duodenal papilla and may be
F released together.

G 1 Heptic ducts L = left / R = right

H 2 Common hepatic duct

I 3 Heister's valve

J 4 GB duct

K 5 Common bile duct

L 6 Pancreatic duct

M 7 opening of the pancreatic duct
      (into the common bile duct)

N 8 Major duodenal papilla = Papilla of Vater
      (in the descending duodenum)

O 9 LN in the duodenum

P 10 Plicae circulares of the Duodenum

Q 11 Serosa – capsule of the GB

R 12 Fundus of the GB

S 13 Mucosa

T 14 folds in the GB

   15 body of the GB - *site of gall stones - note no pain here
U   only when small stones try to pass down the duct.

V 16 neck of the GB

W *Gallstones – biliary calculi, solidification of the bile made up of its
   components, bile pigment, calcium salts, cholesterol present in 10% of
X the population.

Y

Z

© A. L. N

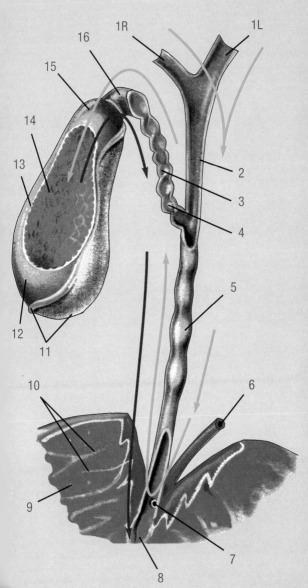

1R

1L

16

15

14

13

2

3

4

5

6

12

11

10

9

8

7

Gall Bladder –
Cystic duct & Cystic artery relations

schematic – anterior
cystic artery posterior to the cystic duct
cystic artery anterior to the cystic duct

Description: the gall bladder (GB) is supplied by the cystic artery which ~1/2 the time, arises from the R hepatic artery and half the time from the Proper hepatic artery.

The artery runs deep to the cystic duct also ½ the time.

CALOT'S triangle – locates the cystic artery – it is bounded by the inf surface of the liver – the cystic duct & the body of the GB.

On palpation the artery has a pulse and the duct if stressed will initiate a peristaltic movement.

1 Hepatic ducts L = left / R = right
2 Common hepatic duct
3 Common bile duct
4 Cystic duct
5 GB = vesica biliaris b = body / n = neck
6 Proper hepatic a
7 Coeliac trunk
8 Hepatic arteries L = left / R = right
9 Cystic a

© A. L. Ne

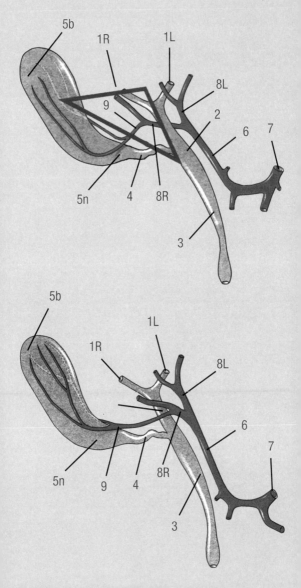

Gall Bladder – duct variations

The bile ducts and their relations with each other and ducts from associated organs – in particular -the pancreas have a number of common variations – this is important surgically as the GB is often removed.

Cystic duct

ventral view – normal cystic duct pathway
ventral view – spiral cystic duct pathway

Description: The cystic duct generally travels inferiorly before joining the common Hepatic duct and forming the common bile duct. However in some cases (15-20%) it spirals ventrally in front of the Common hepatic duct before joining it.

1 Hepatic ducts L = left / R = right

2 Common hepatic duct

3 Duodenum 1st part

4 junction b/n cystic & common hepatic ducts forming the...

5 Common bile duct

6 Pancreatic duct

7 2nd part of the duodenum

8 GB

9 Cystic duct

10 Inf. edge of the liver

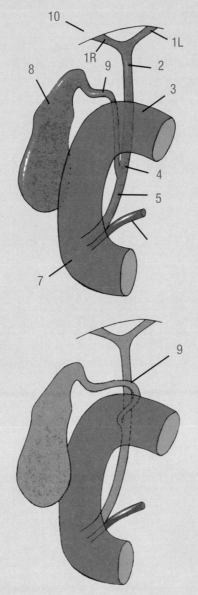

Genioglossus - 1

O	superior mental spine of symphysis menti (mandibular symphysis)
I	ventral surface of the central mass of tongue and its mucous membrane interdigitating with intrinsic muscles of the tongue
	hypoglossal membrane and the upper anterior surface of the hyoid interdigitates with the superior pharyngeal constrictor
A	protracts tongue / pokes out tongue
	depression of the centre of the tongue to form a tunnel
NS	C1 travelling + hypoglossal N (CN XII)
BS	facial – lingual branches
T	ability to poke out tongue
	ability to curl up tongue into a tube/tunnel

Geniohyoid - 2

This muscle partially determines the chin line drawing a line b/n the Mandible and the Hyoid

O	inferior mental spine posterior of symphysis menti (mandibular symphysis)
I	anterior surface of hyoid
A	elevation and protrusion of Hyoid
	depression of mandible (fixed hyoid)
NS	C1 travelling with hypoglossal N (CN XII)
BS	facial – mandibular branch
T	observe swallowing
	open jaw against R

Both these muscles are - as are all muscles of the tongue - involved in the movement of food around the mouth to facilitate chewing and position the food bolus for swallowing.

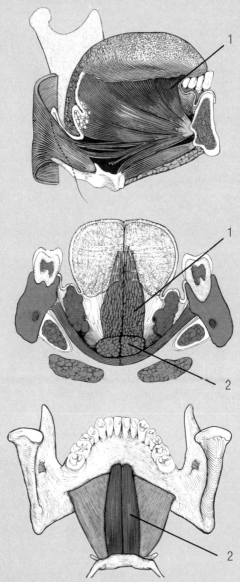

Hiatus Hernia - Oesophagus

A
B *Schematic*

C **Description:** the oesophagus passes through the diaphragm at the
D oesophageal hiatus – where it is connected to the diaphragm via
the the phrenico-oesophageal ligament = Laimer's membrane. The
E R crus of the diaphragm and the circular fibres of the Cardia act
as physiological sphincter and valve to prevent backflow from the
F stomach. This is helped by the angle created when the
G oesophagus abruptly enters the stomach. – the angle of His.

H Hiatus hernias occur with loosening of the ligament and widening
of the orifice - allowing the stomach to prolapsed into the thorax.
I Then acid may enter the oesophagus which does not have the
thick mucoid coat to protect it from acid erosion, causing GERD =
J gastro-oesophageal reflux disease = acid reflux = "heartburn"–
K pain in the centre of the chest related to eating ± posture. -

L Axial hernias – widening of the orifice only.

M Sliding hernias – movement of the cardia ± fundus into the thorax
with its peritoneal covering.

N Many hiatal hernias are asymptomatic however if the stomach is
O still acidic - damage is occuring.

P   1 Oesophagus – lumen

Q   2 Angle of His – much less acute in infants allowing
          for easier vomiting and regurgitation

R   3 Phrenico-oesophageal lig = Laimers' membrane –
S   reinforced with strong CT fibres

T   4 Diaphragm – muscle L= left crus / R = right crus

U   5 Cardiac orifice (of the stomach)

V   6 Peritoneal cavity

     7 Diaphragmatic fascia I = inferior / s = superior
W
     8 Peritoneal membrane
X
     9 Vestibule
Y
    10 Ampulla
Z
    11 Oesophageal fascia

© A. L. Neill

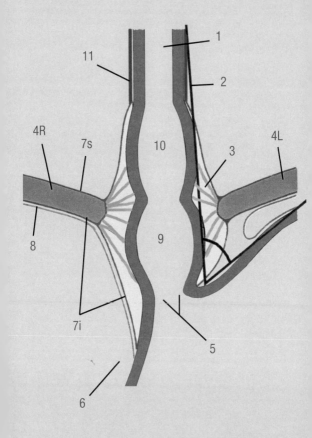

A
Ileocaecal junction

B *Anterolateral - looking onto the DT cavities*

C **Definition:** the point at which the SI becomes the LI. A "valve"
D exists at this point in that flow can be modified and if the caecum
is full – the flow is stopped or delayed, but the 1° function of this
E sphincteric valve is to prevent reflux back to the SI from the LI.*

F 1 Ileocaecal arteries

G 2 smooth muscle layers of the a = ascending colon /
c = caecum / i = ileum / p = appendix (common
H to all in the GIT - outer longitudinal fibres and inner
circular fibres)

J 3 outer serosal layer continuous with the mesentery of
the a = ascending colon / c = caecum / i = ileum /
K p = appendix

L 4 Ileocaecal fold

M 5 Appendicular a – in the appendicular mesentery

N 6 Vermiform appendix (wormlike)

O 7 lumens of the a = ascending colon / c = caecum /
i = ileum / p = appendix

P 8 Semi lunar folds – expanding volume of the caecum

Q 9 Ileocaecal papilla

R 10 Ileocaecal opening & valve –
histology changes here
S

11 Mesentery of the SI p - mesentery of the appendix
T
*note in an endoscopy this point used to determine completion of the
U procedure, this is the site of Vitamin B12 and bile acid absorption.*

V

W

X

Y

Z

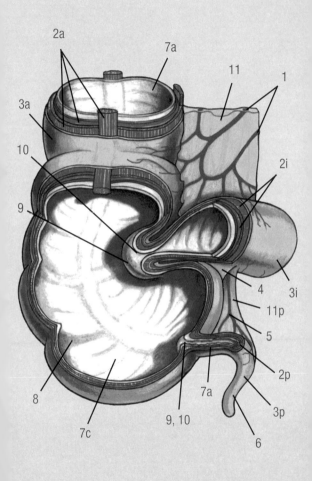

A

Lips – Muscles

B *internal view* - looking into the back of the lips mucosa removed

C *Description:* Muscles of the lips are inserted into the deep fascia,
D and also insert into a common structure the Modiolus.

E 1 Orbicularis oris large circle of muscle around the lips
    L = labial part
F   m = marginal part

G 2 Buccinator

H 3 Modiolus

I 4 Depressor labii inferioris

5 mucous membrane of the lips

J 6 Levator anguli oris

K 7 Incisivus labii superioris

L 8 opening of the oral cavity

M 9 Depressor septi nasi

N
for more details of the bones & muscles see the A to Z of the Head &
O *Neck muscles & bones*

P

Q

R

S

T

U

V

W

X

Y

Z

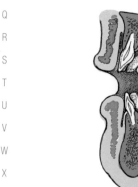

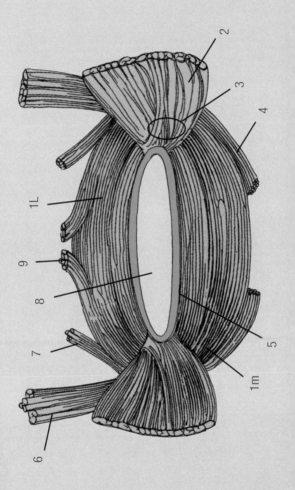

A

Liver

B *Inferior - the liver has been lifted up & is viewed from underneath*

C **Definition:** the liver is the largest organ in the body. It lies in the upper R quadrant, directly under the diaphragm to which it is attached via several ligaments. It moves 1-2 cm with respiration, but is not normally felt below the costal margin. A ptosed liver may indicate CCF, malaria and/or hepatomegaly. This 4 lobed organ has great regenerative powers and generally weighs up to 2kg (4-5lb). It lies on top of several structures, with imprints showing on the inferior surface

1 L coronary lig = appendix fibrosa

2 Gastric imprint

3 Omental tubercle

4 Major lobe of the Liver L = left / R = right

5 Papillary process (of caudate lobe)

6 Caudate lobe – p = process of

7 Inferior margin

8 Hepatic artery c = cystic branch (to the GB)

9 Ligamentum teres = round lig. f = fissure for / n = notch of this is a degenerative lig. from the deterioration of the umbilical bypass vessels in the foetal circulation)

10 Quadrate lobe

11 GB

12 Duodenal imprint

13 Colic imprint

14 Common bile duct

15 Renal imprint

16 Portal vein = Porta Hepatis

17 Coronary lig

18 Suprarenal imprint (of the adrenal gland)

19 Diaphragmatic surface

20 IVC L = ligament of

21 Ligamentum venosum (note covers the degenerative Ligamentum teres)

22 Oesophageal imprint

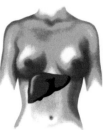

© A. L. Ne

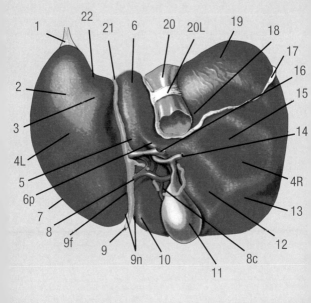

A # Liver

B *Upper – Anterior - schema of the BF*

C *Lower – Posterior - view looking at the back of the liver*

D **Description:** the liver receives the GIT venous blood via the
PORTAL vein. From there it drains to the IVC. The blood flows
E through the liver parenchyma via the sinusoids - open capillaries
which allow for fluid, substance and cell movement into and out of
F the BVs. The arterial supply is via the hepatic artery which also
G drains to the IVC.

H 1 IVC

I 2 R & L hepatic veins

3 capillary network – sinusoids
J
4 cystic duct

K 5 hepatic artery

L 6 common bile duct

M 7 hepatic PORTAL vein

N 8 gall bladder

9 bile duct network
O
10 caudate lobe (BS – R hepatic art and vein)
P
11 R & L lobes of the liver
Q
12 round ligament separating the R & L BS

R 13 quadrate lobe (BS – R hepatic art and vein)

S 14 Porta Hepatis = 5+6+7

T

U

V

W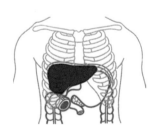

X

Y

Z

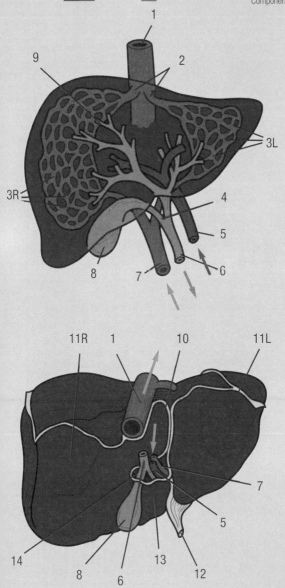

© A. L. Neill

Blood supply of the Liver Venous supply

anterior schematic overview

Definition: the liver is the largest organ in the body. It lies in the upper R quadrant. It is the major detoxifying organ – most of the absorbed material must first pass through this organ before entering the main BS. It also produces bile which assists greatly in fat digestion. In order to facilitate substances entering and leaving hepatocytes (liver cells), specially structured BF arranged in hexagonal lobules and veins – sinusoids – are unique features of this organ. This 4 lobed organ has great regenerative powers and generally weighs up to 2kg (4-5lb).

1 IVC

2 Hepatic vein L= left / R = right

3 Caudate hepatic vein (directly from IVC)

4 Superior hepatic vein L= left / R = right

5 Radial veins (radix veins) I = inferior / S = superior

6 anterior surface of the liver

7 Portal vein

8 distributing veins

9 Sinusoids

10 Central vein

11 Sublobular veins

12 posterior lateral hepatic vein

13 Middle hepatic vein – superficial

A = arterial blood entering the liver – oxygenated

B = bile leaving the liver to digest fat and lipids

P = portal blood from the GIT - deoxygenated nutrient rich

S = blood being detoxified through the sinusoids

V = deoxygenated and detoxified blood returning to the body via the IVC

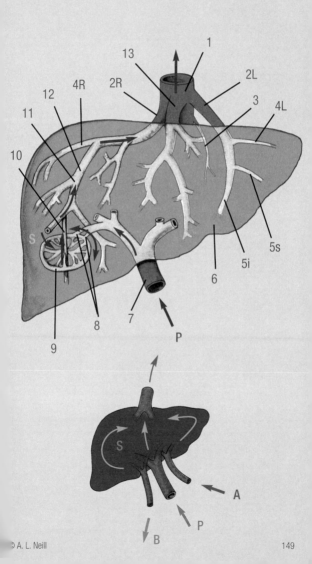

Blood supply of the Liver Sinusoids

Definition: the sinusoid is the specifically modified capillary of the liver. In order for substances to flow in and out with ease. The BM, a protein and fibrous network, and the endothelial cells lining the capillaries have large complete gaps and which allows protein to leave and blood including blood cells to move into the hepatocytes. Flow is slow and LP.

macroscopic schematic overview

1. Hepatic v
2. sinusoid p = peripheral, r = radial
3. interconnecting sinusoids / b/n hepatic lobules
4. venule sphincters i = inlet / o = outlet
5. distributing v
6. branch of Hepatic a
7. branch of Portal v
8. bile ductile
9. liver functioning unit – blood flows from here to the central vein (10)
10. central v
11. sublobular v = interlobular v

A = arterial blood entering the liver – oxygenated
B = bile leaving the liver to digest fat and lipids
P = portal blood from the GIT - deoxygenated nutrient rich
S = blood being detoxified through the sinusoids
V = deoxygenated and detoxified blood returning to the body via the IVC

microscopic schematic overview

1. BM
2. endothelial cell nucleus
3. cytoplasm of the endothelium
4. vacuole for transport of substances
5. RBC
6. cell to cell connection in endothelium
7. fenstration
8. gap in endothelium + BM

© A. L. Nei

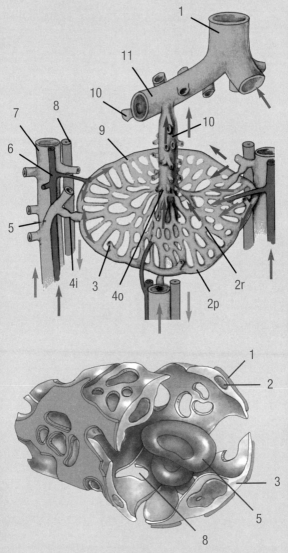

© A. L. Neill

A

Mesentery

B *Schematic*

C *Definition:* the connective tissue fascial layer which surrounds the
D components of the GIT, and acts as the anchor to the posterior
abdominal wall. It is derived from the peritoneum.

E
The stomach, transverse colon, appendix and sigmoid colon all
F have their own mesenteries, the rest of the GIT is fixed to the
posterior wall of the abdomen. The mesentery allows for mobility of
G the gut and improves peristalsis – but it also allows for twisting
and torsion of the gut, which may result in ischaemia and death of
H the twisted sections. Necrosis of the gut may result in perforation
I and release of the contents into the peritoneum – and peritonitis.

J The greater omentum is 2 layers of the peritoneum fused together
– and has a similar structure to mesenteric tissue.

K
1 SI
L
2 Vessels in the mesentery – note there are arteries
M veins and lymphatics

N 3 major art supplying the mesentery
only arteries shown

O
4 connective tissue layer – generally a thin CT
P network with fat spread throughout but may act as a
store for fat and be quite thick in obese patients
Q

R

S

T

U

V

W

X

Y

Z

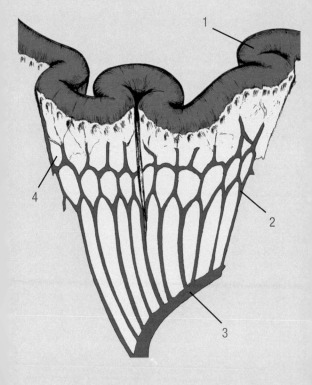

Nose – in situ

Lateral, Medial

Definition: The nose consists of the nasal cavity & the surrounding

structures around that cavity. These are made up of many contributing bones similar to the paranasal sinuses, & other structures such as cartilages.

1 Frontal bone, 1s = Frontal sinus

2 Nasal bone

3 Nasal cartilages – 3L = lateral cartilage
   3A = alar cartilage, 3S = septal cartilage

4 Nostril = nare = nasal opening

5 Lips

6 Maxilla – with tooth embedded

7 Palatine bone (making up the hard palate)

   7i = incisive canal

8 Inferior concha

9 Sphenoid bone

   9L = lateral pterygoid plate 9s = Sphenoid sinus

10 Ethmoid bone
   10c = cribiform plate, 10m = medial concha

   10p = perpendicular plate, 10s = superior concha

11 Sphenopalatine foramen

12 Lacrimal bone

13 Vomer

contribution of the Frontal bone

contribution of the Sphenoid

contribution of the Maxilla

contribution of the Ethmoid bone

inferior nasal concha (is its own bone)

Vomer

Nasal bone

Lacrimal bone

contribution of the Palatine bone

cartilages

*The nasal cartilages are illustrated in detail in the **A to Z of Surface***

Anatomy

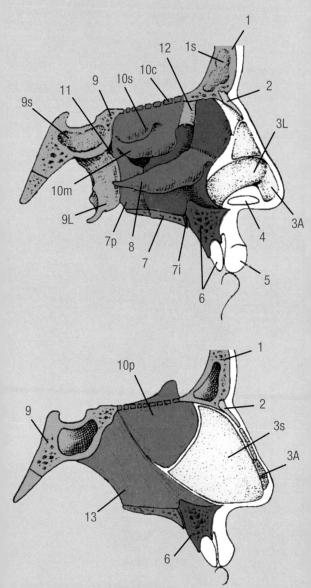

Nose - Blood supply

Lateral view looking at the Conchae / Turbinates
Medial view looking at the Septum

The BS of the nose involves the joining of several BVs which anastomose in the septum and tip. This is a very well supplied area and prone to injury, and changes with hormones and other factors.

1. frontal sinus

2. lat. nasal br of the facial art – to the ala of the nose

3. int. nasal Br from V_2 (infraorbital N)

4. nasal conchae – turbinates
   i = inferior / m = middle / s = superior

5. nasal br of ant palantine N
   (from pterygopalantine ganglion)

6. Pterygoid plate of the Sphenoid

7. sphenopalantine a (from Maxillary)

8. post. ethmoidal a

9. ant ethmoidal a

10. ant ethmoidal N (V_1)

11. cut br of ant ethmoidal N – to tip of nose

12. subseptal a – from superior labial at (upper lip)

13. Hard palate

14. Sphenoidal sinus

15. Nasalpalatine N (from pterygopalantine ganglion)

16. Nasoseptal a (from 7)

17. Ethmoid plate

18. Little's area, site of anastomoses of several BVs - prone to haemorrhage

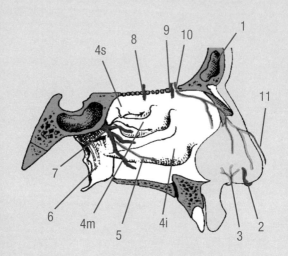

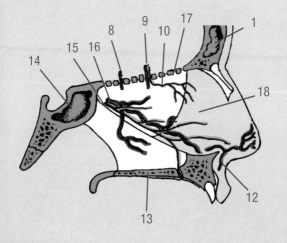

A

Oesophagus

B

Description: The oesophagus connects the mouth with the stomach - mainly in the thorax it passes through the diaphragm to the abdomen and empties its contents. It has considerable room to expand and the mucosal layer has vertical folds to allow this. The upper 1/3 is skeletal muscle which changes to become completely smooth muscle in the lower 1/3. It is lined with a stratified epithelium and has no absorptive funtion.

C

D

E

F

G

1 Epiglottis – the "lid" to stop food going into the Trachea – respiratory system

H

2 Thyroid cartilage

I

3 Cricoid cartilage - point of division b/n trachea & oesophagus

J

K

4 Oesophagus – continuous with the pharynx / throat - commencing at the cricoid cartilage

L

5 Trachea - anteriorly cartilaginous but the posterior wall is muscular allowing for expansion by the oesophagus

M

N

6 Aorta – to the L initially then moves to be posterior - as it enters the heart – note the proximity of the Oesophagus and the heart

O

P

7 Bronchi L= left R = right

Q

8 Muscular layers of the oesophagus – inner circular / outer longitudinal – a pattern common throughout the layers of the GIT

R

S

9 Diaphragm = Cardia

T

10 Cardiac Stomach – so called bc of its proximity to the heart

U

V

11 Abdominal oesophagus – completely smooth muscle layers at this stage

W

12 R Crus of the Diaphragm making up the physiologica sphincter of the oesophagus = oesophageal sphincter.

X

Y

Serosal layer not shown

Z

© A. L. Ne

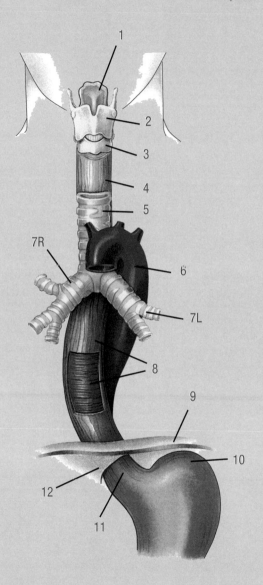

Oesophagus – Nerve Supply

Description: The NS of the oesophagus gradually becomes more automatic with progression down the tube – as does the muscle character change from skeletal muscle to smooth muscle. Its own intrinsic NS acts w/o external stimulation and perpetuates food bolus progression via peristalsis. External modification comes from the Sympathetic trunk and the Vagus N (CN X)

1 Lumen – note vertical rugae/folds

2 Epithelial lining – non keratinized stratified epithelium changing towards the gastric end to – simple columnar epithelium with a few mucous glands – little protection against acid reflux

3 Submucosal plexus = Meissner's plexus part of the intrinsic NS

4 Inner circular layer of muscle (skeletal at the oral end – smooth at the gastric end)

5 Myenteric plexus = Auerbach's plexus part of the intrinsic NS

6 Fascial layer b/n the muscle layers containing collagen and elastic fibres

7 Outer longitudinal layer of muscle

8 Submucosal layer

9 Thin muscle layer = muscularis mucosa

Serosal layer not shown

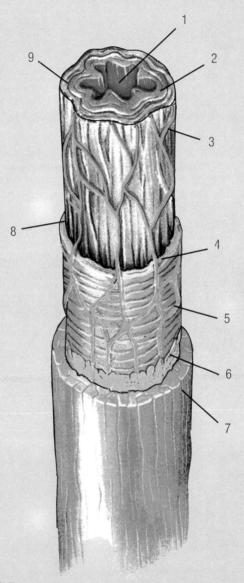

Oesophagus – Blood Supply & Lymphatic drainage

Description: The oesophagus connects the mouth with the stomach - the base is a site where the portal BS - LP is mixed with the systemic BS - HP. In portal hypertension the B from the L gastric vein to the Azygos aas and submucosal varicosities develop - oesophageal varicosities, which are fragile vessels subject to bleeding. Serious anaemia or even shock may develop from unchecked bleeding from these BVs.

1. Cricoid cartilage*
2. Oesophageal a from inf. thyroid a
3. Aortic arch + level of tracheal bifurcation*
4. Oesophageal brs. from the thoracic aorta
5. level of L atrium – expanded in mitral stenosis – causing oesophageal constriction pathological
6. level of entry to the abdomen through the diaphragm - causing oesophageal constriction pathological
7. Oesophageal br from the splenic a
8. Fundus of the stomach
9. Oesophageal br from the L gastric a
10. Oesophageal br from the inf phrenic a
11. Aorta emerging into the abdomen through the diaphragm
12. Gastric veins L = left / R = right
13. Hepata portis = hepatic portal v
14. Oesophageal brs of the gastric veins & gastric LNs
15. IVC
16. Inf. phrenic vein & oesophageal brs + inf phrenic LNs
17. Azygos v + oesophageal brs – near prevertebral LNs (post.)
18. intercostal brs drain to the Azygos
19. oesophageal LNs
20. SVC
21. Paratracheal LNs
22. Supraclavicular LNs
23. Deep cervical LNs
24. Inf. thyroid v + oesophageal brs

*an oesophageal constriction

Oesophageal carcinomas spread early and extensively because of the extensive LN network around this organ.

© A. L. Nei

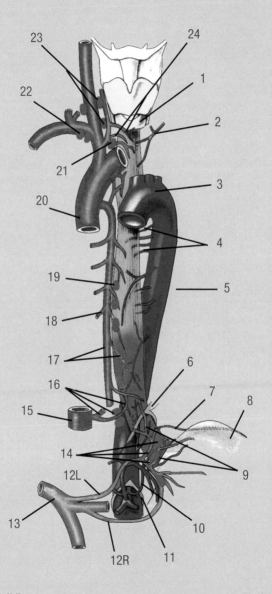

Omental Bursa

Sagittal cut – with anterolateral view to show spatial relationships

Definition: spaces created in the abdominal region by the folding of the mesenteries & omenta

Description: as the mesentery develops and folds with growth of the GIT organs, it creates closed areas. An understanding of these spaces – bursa allows for access to all areas in the peritoneal cavity w/o compromising any BS. Inflammation in the abdominal cavity often causes adhesions in the greater omentum and to many of the abdominal organs.

1 Hepatogastric lig. of the Lesser omentum
2 Lesser sac of the omental bursa
3 Post. peritoneal layer
4 Stomach
5 Splenic a & v
6 Pancreas
7 Gastrocolic lig.
8 Transverse mesocolon = mesentery of the transverse colon
9 Transverse colon
10 Greater sac of the omental bursa
11 Greater omentum - d = dorsal layer / v =ventral layer
12 Omental BVs
13 Hepatic flexure of the colon = R colic flexure
14 R gastroepiploic BVs
15 GB
16 Pyloris + superior part of the Duodenum
17 proper hepatic a
18 Falciform lig (containing ligamentum teres = round lig)
19 R and L lobes of the liver

note – when referring to the abdomen – often the terms ventral /dorsal replace anterior / posterior

2 + 10 = the omental bursa

3 common access points through the: lesser omentum (i), gastrocolic lig (ii) and the transverse mesocolon (iii).

© A. L. Neil

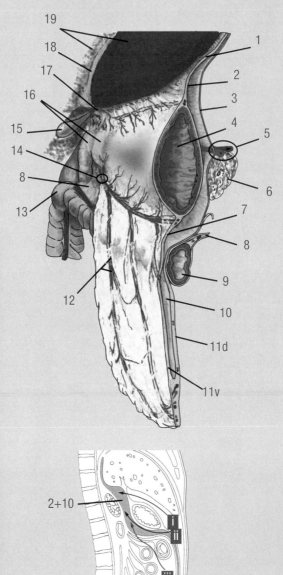

19
18
17
16
15
14
8
13

1
2
3
4
5
6
7
8
9
10
11d
11v
12

2+10

i
ii
iii

© A. L. Neill

Omentum – Greater = Greater Omentum

Anterior wall removed

Definition: from Lt Omental = Apron

Description: One of 2 peritoneal folds (also the Lesser Omentum) arising from the greater curvature of the stomach falling over the anterior of the abdomen and its contents – and then folding back to reattach to the stomach. Full of fatty lymphoid and vascular elements; it acts as a shield and bandage to the gut contents. Injured parts of the gut may be isolated and sealed by this freely moving tissue sheet. It is also a storage of fat and responsible in part for the "Beer gut."

1 Diaphragm

2 Spleen

3 Stomach

4 Greater curvature of the stomach and omental attachment

5 Urinary bladder

6 SI

7 Greater omentum – fat globules

8 Greater omentum BVs and Lymphatic tissue

9 GB

10 Liver – L lobe

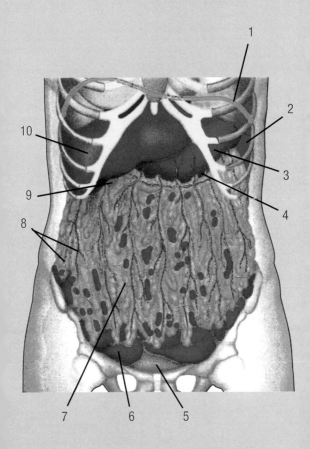

Pancreas

Anterior – cutaway to demonstrate the path of the duct

Description: the pancreas is a grey "comma-shaped" organ up to 15cm long, fixed ot the posterior abdominal wall - lying in the upper abdomen and extending from the R – where its head inserts into the "C" of the duodenum – to the L where its tail extends into the hilus of the spleen.

It is both an exocrine and endocrine gland. It produces digestive enzymes. These are secreted via the serous glands into the pancreatic duct which travels to the descending duodenum. It also produces hormones into the BS - most importantly INSULIN and GLUCAGON from its endocrine islets (islets of Langerhans). Because of its sweet taste it was referred to as a "sweetmeat" and eaten as a delicacy.

1 Common bile duct

2 Tale of the pancreas

3 Body of the pancreas

4 Pancreatic duct

5 Head of the pancreas

6 Opening – common to the pancreatic duct and common bile duct –
   note this appears as a papilla in the mucosa of the duodenum = Duodenal papilla

7 Pancreatic sphincter = Sphincter of Oddi

8 Accessory pancreatic duct – present in 30%

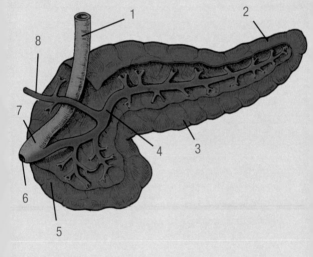

Pancreas – Blood supply

posterior - Arterial supply from the posterior aspect

Description: the pancreas is intimately related to the spleen and duodenum and this is reflected in the BS.

1 Spleen
2 L gastroepiploic a
3 Short gastric a
4 Splenic a
5 Dorsopancreatic a
6 Coelic trunk
7 Common hepatic a
8 L & R Hepatic a
9 common bile duct a
10 Proper hepatic a
11 Supraduodenal a
12 Gastroduodenal a
13 R gastroepiploic a
14 Superior pancreato duodenal a
15 aas – branches
16 Duodenum – posterior surface
17 Anterior br (of the splenic a)
18 Post br
19 Inf. pancreato duodenal a
20 Superior mesenteric a
21 Inf. pancreatic a
22 Great pancreatic a
23 Pancreas – post aspect

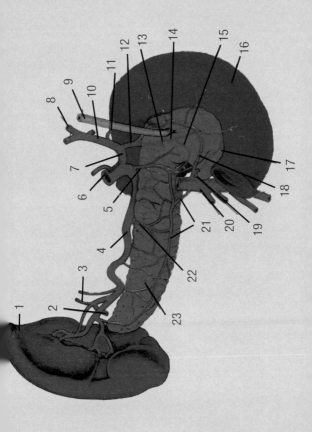

A **Pancreas – Blood supply**

B *posterior* - Venous supply from the posterior aspect

C *Description:* the pancreas is intimately related to the spleen and
D duodenum and this is reflected in the BS. The Venous supply
varies from the arterial as indicated but many aspects are
E mirrored.

F 1 Short gastric vessels
G 2 Splenic - in the groove on post surface of pancreas
3 Portal v
H 4 Common bile duct
I 5 Superior pancreato-duodenal veins
J 6 R gastroepiploic v
K 7 Duodenum post. surface
L 8 Inf. pancreato-duodenal v
M 9 Superior mesenteric v
10 Inferior mesenteric – note drains to the splenic v
N 11 Pancreatic brs
O 12 L gastroepiploic v
P 13 Multiple veins from the splenic hilum

Q

R

S

T

U

V

W

X

Y

Z

© A. L. Ne.

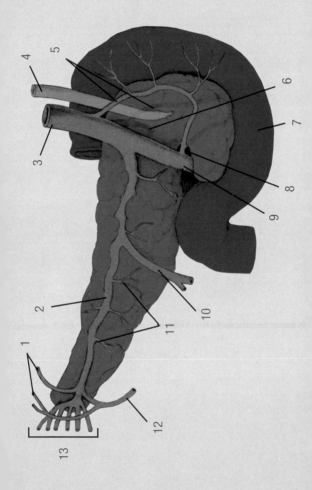

© A. L. Neill

173

Pancreas – necrosis resulting from rupture

Schematic – Sagittal view of pathways of access and damage from a ruptured pancreas

Description: The pancreas is a complex gland which secretes strong proteolytic enzymes. As the organ is retroperitoneal leakage will have access to the entire abdominal region, causing necrosis – in a manner unlike a ruptured gastric ulcer which has the protection of the omenta.

1 Pancreas

2 Liver

3 Stomach + Duodenum

4 Transverse colon

5 SI

6 Greater Omentum

7 Outer peritoneal wall

8 Bladder

9 Sigmo-colon junction - beginning of the sigmoid colon

10 Rectum

a – spillage into the omental bursa

b – spillage into the transverse mesocolon

c – spillage into the root of the mesentery (of the SI)

d – spillage into retroperitoneal space

e – spillage into the false pelvis and inguinal region

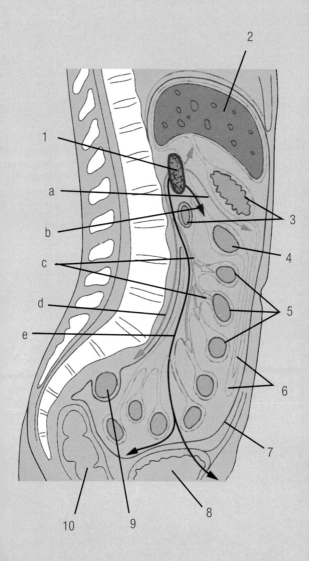

Pancreatic duct variations

Schematic

Description: the 2 major ducts entering the duodenum can do so in various ways. The major variations are shown here.

Because of the intimate relations between the head of the pancreas and the common bile duct - painless jaundice may be the 1st sign of a pancreatic carcinoma

1 Common bile duct

2 Duodenum - 2nd part

3 Accessory pancreatic duct = duct of Santorini - enters directly through minor duodenal papilla only (10%), joins the main pancreatic duct (30%) - 2 entrances
or only enters via the main pancreatic duct (70%)

4 Hepatopancreatic orifice (s) ducts may be separated by a septum – or joint opening for both ducts

5 Major duodenal papilla = Duodenal papilla = Vater's papilla

6 Common pancreatic duct = duct of Wirsung

7 Head of Pancreas

8 Brünner's glands = duodenal glands – alkaline mucous glands of the duodenum in the Submucosa

9 Pancreas tail

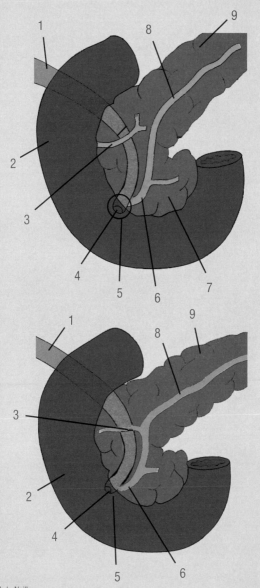

Salivary glands –
Parotid, Submandibular

Lateral view – skin and subcutaneous fat cut away

Description: The parotid gland lies next to the ear - it can become clinically significant if it enlarges as it is close to the Facial N (CN VII) - which innervates most of the muscles of the face and carotid artery - giving the person a swollen face appearance.

The appearance of a Bell's palsy may indicate a parotid gland tumour. Dry mouth from reduced salivary secretion as in autoimmune wasting diseases of the salivary glands may cause increased dental decay and xerostomia.

1 Subcutaneous fat

2 Parotid gland

3 Accessory parotid gland (present in 30%)

4 Parotid duct

5 Modiolus – meeting point of muscles of the face

6 Mylohyoid m

7 deep facial fascia

8 Submandibular gld

9 Mandible – Jaw

10 Masseter m

11 Sternocleidomastoid –SCM

for more details of the bones & muscles see the A to Z of the Head & Neck bones & muscles

© A. L. Ne

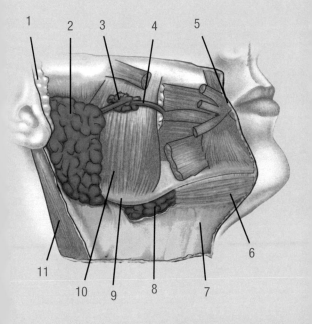

Peritoneal cavity – Peritoneum

Sagittal view

Description: The peritoneum is the 2 layered fascial bag which forms the peritoneal cavity. The outer layer – parietal peritoneum – lines the abdominal cavity. The inner layer – visceral peritoneum – supports the BS & NS of its contents forming various mesenteries and ligaments to do so.

1. Hepatogastric lig. of the lesser omentum
2. Liver
3. Epiploic foramen (of Winslow)
4. Stomach
5. Transverse mesocolon + Transverse colon
6. Greater omentum – showing 4 layers of mesentery and space b/n *
7. Root of mesentery + SI
8. Peritoneal cavity
9. Bladder (outside peritoneum)
10. Anus
11. border – to rectum – leaving peritoneal cavity
12. Sigmoid colon
13. Retroperitoneal space
14. Duodenum – (horizontal = 3rd part)
15. Pancreas
16. bare area of the liver – abuts the diaphragm

*note these layers may fuse in later life or after injury or surgery

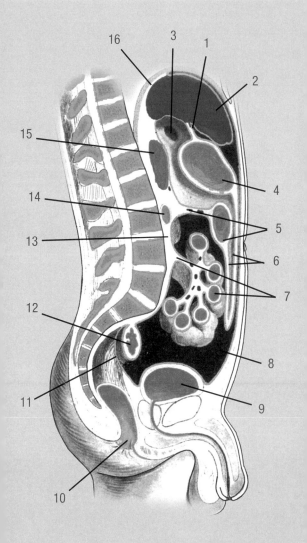

Peritoneal cavity

Transverse view — level of L2

Description: The peritoneal cavity is a mesentery separate bag

containing most of the GIT. Its inner wall supports their BVs with
mesenteries and its outer wall covers those organs which are

outside the cavity. It is a separate space w/in the abdominal cavity.

1 Gastrocolic lig. of the lesser omentum

2 Liver

3 Kidney + perirenal fat

4 Stomach

5 Transverse mesocolon + Transverse colon

6 Greater omentum + bursa

7 Root of mesentery + SI

8 Peritoneal cavity

9 Bladder (outside peritoneum)

10 R colic flexure

11 border — to rectum — leaving peritoneal cavity

12 Descending colon

13 Retroperitoneal space

14 Duodenum — (horizontal = 3rd part)

15 Pancreas

16 Abdominal aorta + IVC

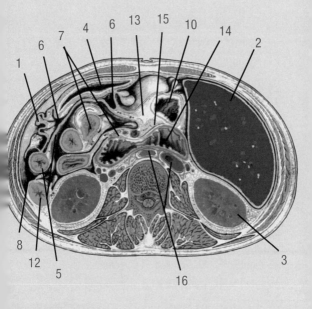

A
Pharynx – overview
B *Posterior – schematic intact*

C *Posterior – divided constrictor muscles*

D *Description:* The pharynx (part of the throat) is that area at the
back of the mouth – 12cm (5 ins) long, extending down the neck
E and in the shape of an inverted cone. It connects the mouth with
the oesophagus. Elevating the soft palate closes the nasopharynx
F in swallowing, so stopping the food coming out of the nose.
G Sneezing occurs when this closure becomes uncoordinated.

H   1 Skull

I   2 Adenoid tonsil

   3 Soft palate

J   4 Phayngeal constrictors i = inf /m = middle/ s = superior

K   5 Epiglottis

L   6 laryngeal inlet

   7 Cricoid cartilage

M   8 Oesophageal mucosa – continuous with oral mucosa

N   9 Oesophagus

O 10 Piriform fossa and opening to oesophagus

  11 Oral mucosa – continues throughout the pharynx

P 12 Tonsil

Q 13 Uvula

R 14 Orophayngeal isthmus

  15 Palato-pharyngeal fold

S 16 Nasal choane = turbinates

T 17 Nasal septum

U 18 Thyroid gland

  19 Parathyroid glands

V 20 Tracheal cartilage

W 21 Hyoid

X   A = NASO-PHARYNX

       B = ORO-PHARYNX

Y   C= LARYNGO-PHARYNX

Z   A + B + C = Pharynx

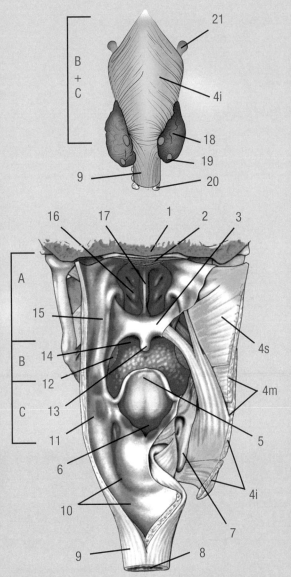

A Rectum & Anal Canal
B Blood Supply – Arterial

C *Description:* The arterial supply of the rectum and anal canal like
D the facial vessels is richly anastomotic – particularly at the anorectal junction.

E
1 Aorta

F
2 L colic a

G
3 Sigmoid a

H
4 Ext. iliac a

I
5 Int. iliac a

J
6 Pudendal a

7 Anal canal + recto arterial plexus & anastomoses

K
8 Pelvic diaphragm

L
9 Inf. rectal a

M
10 Middle rectal a

N
11 Rectum

O
12 Superior rectal a

P
13 Inf mesenteric a

Q
14 IVC

R

S

T

U

V

W

X

Y

Z

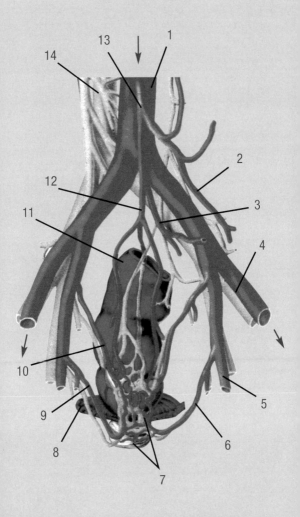

Rectum & Anal Canal
Lymphatic drainage & Lymph nodes

Description: The lymphatic drainage of the rectum and anal canal is intimately related to the pelvic and inguinal lymphatic drainage. Infections &/or neoplasms in these areas spread rapidly because of this highly branched and interconnected network.

1. Aorta + Para-aortic LNs (= Lateral aortic LNs)
2. Inf mesenteric a
3. Sigmoid a
4. Middle rectal art + rectal LNs
5. Int. iliac art + iliac LNs
6. Pudenal art + LNs
7. Pelvic diaphragm
8. LNs connecting to the superficial inguinal LN networks
9. Inf. rectal LNs
10. Coccygeal LNs – post. to the Rectum
11. Sacral LNs – post. to the Rectum
12. Rectum + Para-rectal LNs
13. Superior rectal a + superior rectal LNs
14. Common iliac LNs – medial, lateral & subaortic

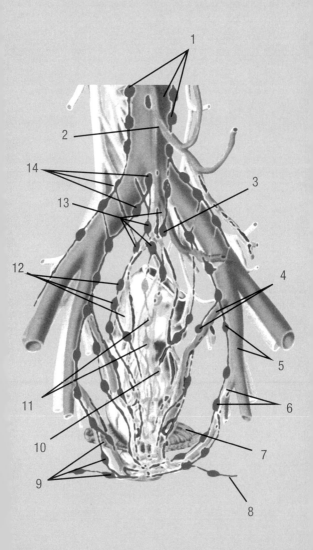

A Rectum & Anal Canal

B Blood Supply – Venous

Description: The venous supply of the rectum and anus is particularly important. It is one of the sites where the LP - low resistance portal venous system meets the HP - high resistance systemic circulation. Any build up of pressure in the portal system will result in the ballooning and expansion of the thin-walled portal veins. This results in Hemorrhoids, which form along the dentate line and may protrude through the anal opening.

1. brs from the SI to the Superior Mesenteric V
2. R Colic V
3. Common Iliac V
   3e – external iliac V
   3i - internal iliac V
4. Sigmoid V
5. Rectal veins
   5i – inferior rectal V
   5m – middle rectal V
   5s - superior rectal V
6. Internal pudendal V
7. Pelvic Diaphragm
8. Anal canal
9. Recto-venous plexus = Porto-venous anastomosis
10. Rectum
11. IVC

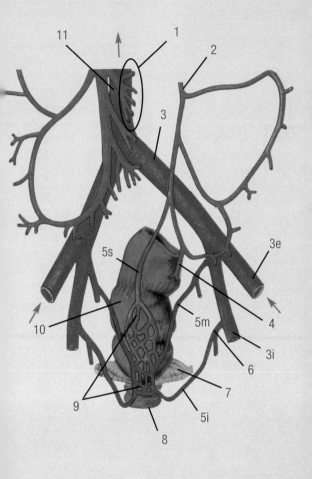

Salivary Glands – in situ

Schematic – open mouth - cutaway to expose the salivary glands and their relationships

Description: The salivary glands have close relations with many other facial structures - e.g. the Facial N & artery and the internal carotid artery. They are essential for digestion and dental health. Of the 3 glands - the parotid is the biggest and the one with the most serous glandular material responsible for producing ptyalin (amylase) an enzyme involved in digestion of carbohydrates. The other glands - produce equal amounts of serosal and mucosal secretions. Saliva is also antiseptic helping in the defense of the oral cavity.

1 Maxilla
2 Incisor tooth
3 Sublingual glands + Frenulum
4 Buccal surface of the gums (Gingiva)
5 pool of saliva
6 Sublingual caruncle - + opening of the Submandibular gland
7 Sublingual gland + ducts – note many small ducts
8 Submandibular duct
9 Submandibular glands – note the 2 parts to the gland around Mylohyoid
10 Mylohyoid m
11 saliva
12 Masseter m
13 Buccinator m
14 Parotid duct
15 Parotid glds
16 Uvula (of the soft palate)
17 Mucous glds of the Palate
18 Hard Palate
19 Tongue
20 Root of tooth in alveolar bone of the Maxilla

A B C D E F G H I J K L M N O P Q R **S** T U V W X Y Z

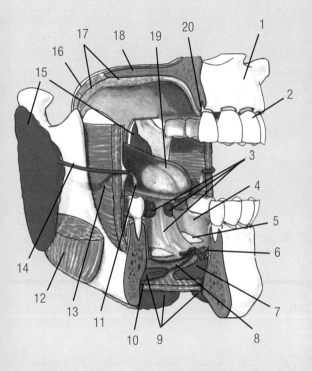

Salivary glands – microscopic overview

Schematic – in situ - showing the microscopic glandular structure within the glands

Description: The sublingual and submandibular glands have 2 types of glands in their structure in approx equal proportions – mucous and serous glands – the content of the cells vary and their ducts but the structure of both is the same. The parotid by far the biggest of all the glands is mainly composed of serous glands which produce enzymes to help with digestion of CHOs. Mucoid secretions are mainly to lubricate the food for easier swallowing.

1 Frenulum of tongue

2 Parotid duct

3 Parotid gland a = accessory gland

4 Submandibular gland

5 Submandibular duct

6 Sublingual gland

7 Sublingual ducts

8 Opening of the submandibular glands

9 Collecting ducts of the glands

10 Duct from the glands

11 Acina of the glands – with saliva present – concentrated as it travels in the collecting ducts before release

12 Glandular cells – producing mucous or ptyalin = amylase – enzyme to digest CHOs

also has an antiseptic property

13 absorbing tubular cells water is resorbed here concentrating the saliva. So slower flowing saliva is stronger than saliva produced in response to food, and water is conserved.

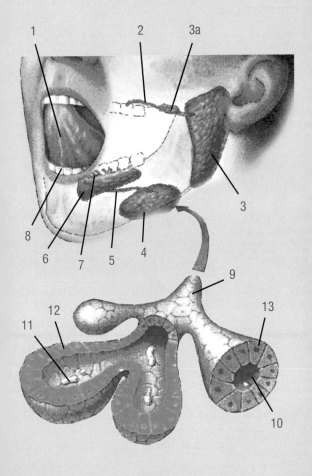

A
Salivary glands – Sublingual,
B
Submandibular
C
*Medial view sagittal section – mucosa and tongue removed
D
looking onto the jaw from the inside*

E
Description: The sublingual and submandibular glands are the 2
smaller salivary glands both mixed mucous and serosal about 50:50
F
each. They lie beneath the tongue and jaw respectively. The
submandibular gland has 2 major parts and like the parotid gland
G
has a major duct opening below the tongue. The sublingual opens in
H
many small ducts along the jaw so is not susceptible to blockages

I
  1 Coronoid process – part of Temporalis attachment
J
  2 Ramus of the Mandible
K
  3 Sublingual gland & small ducts – mucosa stripped away

  4 Gingiva – gums
L
  5 Oral mucosa
M
  6 Submandibular duct
N
  7 Subcutaneous fat + skin
O
  8 Superficial muscles of the face –
     Orbicularis oris + Mentalis
P
  9 Mandible
Q
  10 Mylohyoid m
R
  11 Hyoid

S
  12 Submandibular gland – closely related to the facial
      art (not shown)
T
  13 Angle of the jaw
U
  14 Condylar process – part of the TMJ
V

W
*for more details of the bones & muscles see the A to Z of the Head &
Neck bones & muscles*
X

Y

Z

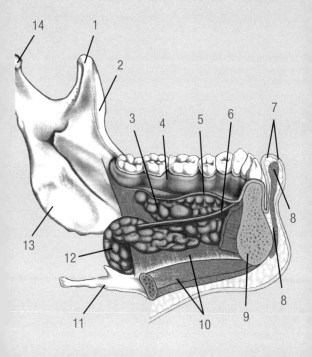

A
Small Intestine – structure

B **Definition:** The GIT b/n the Duodenum to the Caecum, so-called
C due to its small lumen in comparison to the "large intestine." It is
attached to the posterior abdominal wall via a mesentery. It is
D highly mobile and has a very rich BS, and is generally divided into
2 parts. The 1st 1/3 is the jejunum and the latter 2/3 the ileum -
E transition b/n the 2 sections is gradual.

F Sometimes the duodenum is also included - this structure is fixed.

G 1 Serosa – outer layer containing BVs and CT

H 2 Outer longitudinal layer of smooth muscle

I 3 Inner layer of circular of smooth muscle *

J 4 Submucosa

K 5 Mucosa containing..

6 Villi

L 7 lymphoid tissue of the GIT = GALT
M in follicles – lymphoid follicles = Peyer's patches

N 8 Basement membrane

O 9 Muscularis mucosa – inner circular & outer
longitudinal smooth muscle layer

P
10 Plicae circularis – structural fold of the mucosa -
Q unique to the SI formed from LP

R *myenteric N plexus lies b/n these layers and forms part of the intrinsic
NS of the GIT – responsible in part for peristalsis.
S submucosal N plexus b/n the muscle layers in the submucosa.

T

U

V

W

X

Y

Z

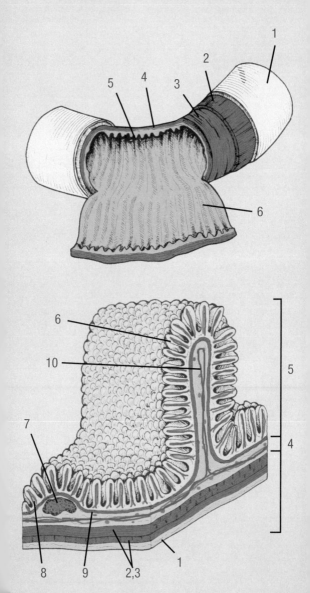

Small Intestine – structure Comparison b/n Jejunum & Ileum

Ileum

Description: The Jejunum is the proximal 1/3 of the SI which slowly changes to the Ileum the remaining 2/3. As the function changes from primarily absorption to that of preparation and storage – with more intestinal flora present, the structure also undergoes changes – summarized below.

features	*Jejunum*	*Ileum*
BVs / BF	*straight large anastomotic loops few branches in the vessels – v vascular – v slow flowing*	*short branched vessels (1) - less vascular - faster flow*
lumen – shape/wall thickness/fat	*single LNs or small follicules (2)*	*smaller - round/thinner*
lymphoid tissue	*single LNs or small follicules (2)*	*extensive - Peyer's patches (3) = large active follicules*
mesentery (4)	*thin - v vascular*	*thick – may contain a lot of fat (4f)*
pH villi (5)	*alkaline* *higher more convoluted – few mucous cells – Plicae Circulares (6) fixed folds to increase surface area*	*alkaline/neutral* *lower – less folds more mucous cells – smaller surface area*

* *Terminal 1/3 of the ileum along with the colon is the commonest site of Crohn's disease lesions, which may involve the whole wall but skip whole areas.*

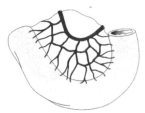

© A. L. Neil

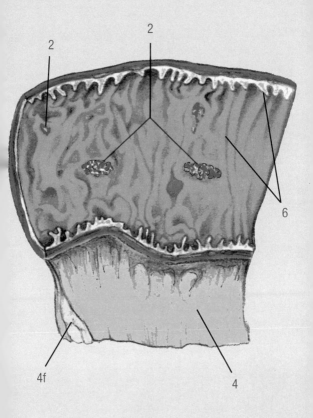

2

2

2

6

4f

4

Small Intestine – structure Comparison b/n Jejunum & Ileum

Jejunum

Description: The Jejunum is the proximal 1/3 of the SI which slowly changes to the Ileum the remaining 2/3. As the function changes from primarily absorption to that of preparation and storage – with more intestinal flora present the structure also undergoes changes – summarized below.

features	Jejunum	Ileum
BVs / BF	straight large anastomotic loops few branches in the vessels – v vascular – v slow flowing	short branched vessels (1) - less vascular - faster flow
lumen – shape/wall thickness/fat	single LNs or small follicules (2)	smaller - round/thinner
lymphoid tissue	single LNs or small follicules (2)	extensive - Peyer's patches (3) = large active follicules
mesentery (4)	thin - v vascular	thick – may contain a lot of fat (4f)
pH	alkaline	alkaline/neutral
villi (5)	higher more convoluted – few mucous cells – Plicae Circulares (6) fixed folds to increase surface area	lower – less folds more mucous cells – smaller surface area

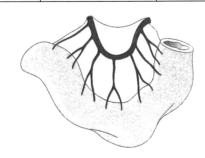

© A. L. Ne

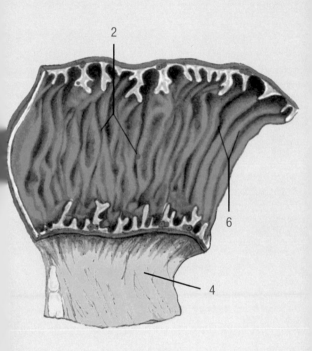

Stomach, Duodenum & Pancreas – Lymphatic Drainage

Description: As with all structures along the GIT, the Stomach and Duodenum have an extensive lymphatic drainage, which is intimately related to the other supportive structures of the region and lies in the mesentery following the BS and draining to the Thoracic duct

1 Cardiac oesophagus and LNs

2 L gastric LNs

3 Diaphragm

4 body of the pancreas and Supra pancreatic LNs

5 Spleen + splenic LNs

6 tail of the pancreas

7 Gastro-omental LNs = gastroepiploic LNS (R & L as with the BS – these are connected with the extensive LNs of the Greater omentum

8 Jejunum

9 Superior mesenteric a + superior mesenteric LNs

10 Aorta and pre-aortic LNs

11 Head of the pancreas

12 Descending duodenum

13 Pylorus + infrapyloric LNs

14 Suprapyloric LNs

15 Superior pancreatic R LNs – connected to the LNs o the Lesser Omentum

16 Cisterna Chyli

17 Coeliac trunk and coeliac LNS

18 Thoracic duct

19 Oesophagus – thoracic

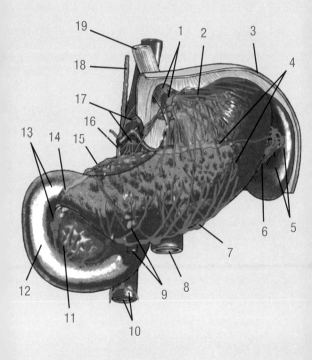

Stomach – position changes and regions

Description: The Stomach is a highly mobile organ. It can contain up to 2 litres of food. The body is not fixed – but the oesophageal and pyloric regions are. The muscle layers of the stomach contract and force the food towards the pyloris whatever its shape making it very functionally very adaptable. Note despite many restrictive surgeries (as in gastric banding) the stomach manages to continue to function well.

Here are examples of 4 different states of a normal stomach.

1 normal

2 actively digesting

3 stretched

4 pregnant*

5 fundus

6 cardia

7 body

8 pylous

A B C D E F G H I J K L M N O P Q R **S** T U V W X Y Z

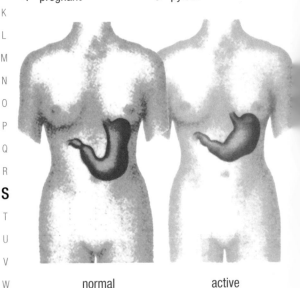

normal   active

It is easy to see why dyspepsia and indigestion is common in pregnancy and obesity.

© A. L. Ne

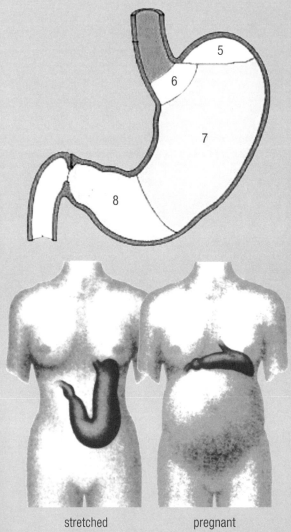

stretched   pregnant

A

Stomach – Blood supply

B *Anterior – in situ – liver removed -*

C *arterial supply mainly demonstrated.*

D *Description:* The stomach is supplied by branches of the coeliac
trunk and has extensive anastomoses on both the lesser and

E greater curves with the joining of the L & R gastric vessels and the
L & R gastroepiploic vessels, and drains via the portal system to

F the liver before entering the IVC.

G
1 Oesophagus coming through the diaphragm

H oesophageal br. of the L gastric a

I
2 Fundus of the stomach

J
3 L gastro-epiploic art

K
4 Short gastric vessels

L
5 Spleen

M
6 Splenic a

N
7 Greater omentum

O
8 Gastro-epiploic R & L aa

P
9 Gastroduodenal a

Q
10 Duodenum + stomach pyloris

R
11 Gall bladder

S
12 Cystic a

13 Portal v + R hepatic duct

T
14 Common hepatic art.

U
15 R gastric a

V
16 Coeliac trunk

W
17 Space in the central tendon of the diaphragm for the IVC

X
18 L gastric a

Y

Z

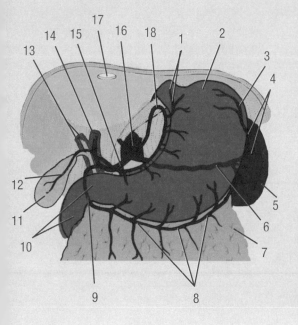

A

Stomach

B *Description:* the stomach is an expandable muscular sac with a highly folded mucosa and acid environment - (pH 1-4) can hold up to 3 litres.

C

D

1   Cardiac oesophagus = Abdominal oesophagus – note vertical mucosal folds

E

2   base of oesophagus - site of oesophageal varicosities

F

3   cardiac notch

G

4   cupola of the stomach

H

5   fundus of stomach - often filled with gas

I

6   folds of the stomach = rugae

J

7   body of the stomach

K

8   curvatures of the stomachs G = greater / L = lesser - sites of omental attachments and major BVS

L

9   serosal layer of the stomach – peritoneal tissue

M

10 multilayered muscular layer of the stomach

N

11 mucosal layer of the stomach – very thick and protective – against the acid environment

O

12 pyloric antrum

P

13 duodenum D = descending part / F = First part

Q

14 Plicae circulares – structural folds of the mucosa exclusive to the duodenum

R

15 pyloric sphincter – rugae of the stomach stream line to the pyloris – contraction of the stomach pushes food into this direction

S

T

16 angular notch

U

17 thickening at the base of the oesophagus – not a sphincter

V

W

X

Y

Z

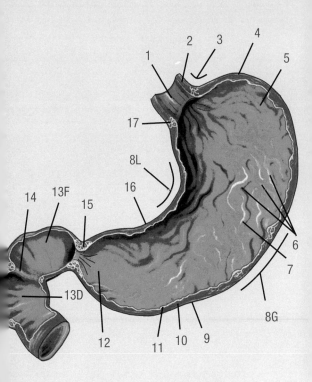

A # **Stomach** – microanatomy

B ## Gastric mucosa

C *Schematic*

D **Description:** The Mucosa = the lining epithelium + the BM + the
loose CT AKA Lamina propria composed of BVS, Lymphoid tissue
E (GALT), and Ns.

F The mucus is very thick due to the acid content of the stomach.
G There are a number of pits which descend into glands, where
Parietal or acid producing cells are found.

H
I 1 heavy mucus coating produced by mucous cells

2 junction b/n glands and gastric pits

J 3 gastric glands – where HCL is produced – note as
K separate ions which combine in the lumen

L 4 capillary

5 muscularis mucosa

M 6 mucous cells

N 7 lamina propria = loose CT below the epithelial lining

O 8 epithelial cells – sitting on the BM

P 9 gastric pits – thick mucus coating – glands below
Q have a thinner coating

R 10 chief cells

S 11 basal cells - move up from the bottom to be
sloughed off on the surface - every 2-3 days

T 12 parietal cells

U

V

W

X

Y

Z

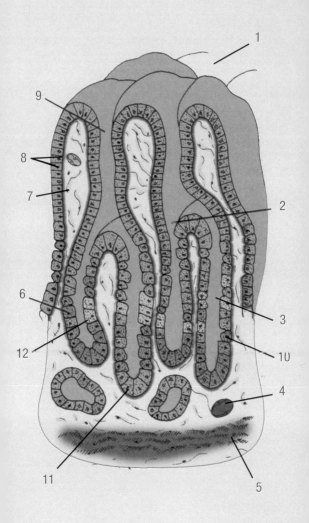

Stomach – Parasympathetic innervation – Vagus (CN X)

Anterior / ventral

Description: the stomach's motility and acid production are primarily controlled externally by the Vagus N (CN X). Vagotomies were a common procedure to reduce the acid production in the stomach and cure / prevent ulcers and acid reflux. Lateral N responsible for motility in the antrum were preserved. Stomach ulcers are now treated mainly by modern pharmacological ulcer therapy.

1 Oesophagus

2 Vagus
  a = Anterior Vagal trunk = R V agus
  p = Posterior Vagal trunk = L Vagus

3 angle of His

4 ant. Gastric Ns

5 ant. Antral N = ant. Gastric br of ant. Vagal trunk

6 post. Antral N = post. Gastric br of post. Vagal trunk

7 superior mesenteric brs

8 pyloric brs

9 coeliac brs

10 Duodenum

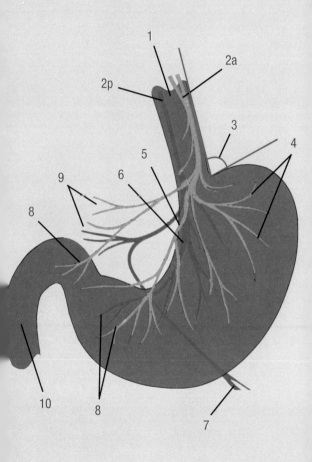

Stomach – muscle layers

Deep

1 Cardiac oesophagus = Abdominal oesophagus – note vertical mucosal folds

2 Longitudinal muscles of the oesophagus

3 deep oblique fibres of the stomach = innermost layer –this is an additional layer

4 fundus of the stomach = gastric fundus

5 curvatures of the stomach G = greater* / L = lesser#

6 submucosa

7 antrum to pyloric region

8 pyloric canal

9 longitudinal muscles of the duodenum

10 pyloris

11 circular layer of oesophagus – continues to the middle muscle layer of the stomach - acts as a "collar" to prevent backflow

#gastric ulcers here may be carcinogenic
* site of most gastric ulcers due to mucosal erosion

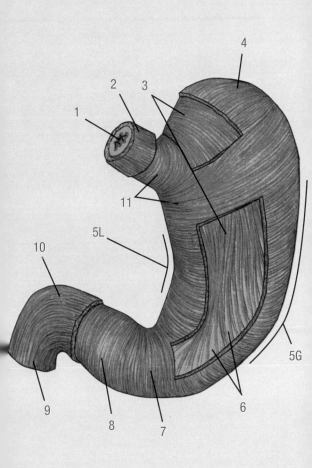

A

Stomach – muscle layers

B *Superficial*

C 1 Cardiac oesophagus = Abdominal oesophagus –
D   note vertical mucosal folds

E 2 Longitudinal muscles of the oesophagus

   3 Cardiac insura = cardiac notch

F 4 External longitudinal fibres of the stomach = outer
G   layers – this is an additional layer only found on the
H   curvatures

I 5 Curvatures of the stomachs G = greater* /
   L = lesser#

J 6 Angular notch = incisure

K 7 Antrum to pyloric region

L 8 Pyloric canal

M 9 Longitudinal muscles of the duodenum

N 10 Pyloris

O 11 Middle circular muscle layer of the stomach

P # gastric ulcers here may be carcinogenic

*site of most gastric ulcers due to mucosal erosion

Q Note: the muscle layers are so arranged as to push the food chyme
R towards the pyloris where, when small enough, it will be forced through

S

T

U

V

W

X

Y

Z

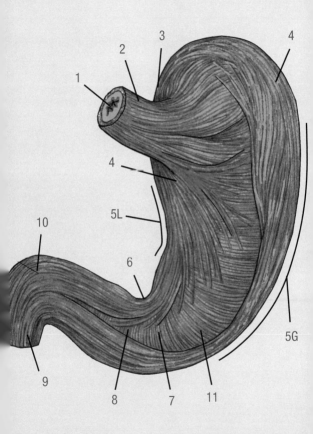

Teeth – permanent dention
normal occlusion

Lateral/Transverse = horizontal crossection just below the gum line

The image of an aligned or correct "bite" = normal occlusion
note the interdigitations b/n the teeth
Common malocclusions
OVERBITE = the upper teeth protrude over the lower,
UNDERBITE = the lower teeth protrude over the upper

This may involve the teeth ± the upper & lower jaws – Maxilla & Mandible.

The bone surrounding the teeth is very thin on the labially (directly under the lips) accounting for the ease with which teeth become dislocated from anterior assaults (punches to the mouth)

C = canine   I = incisor   P = premolar   M = molar

showing crown, neck and roots of each tooth type – along with a superior view of the occlusal surface

1 Root – dentine
2 Neck – changing to enamel = level of the gum
3 Root crown – covered in enamel
4 Interdigitation b/n teeth – occlusion
5 Gum generally slightly above the neck....
6 ..but may recede exposing the weaker dentine to erosion
7 Maxilla
8 Widest point of the palate ~3cm
9 Mandible
10 Root canal containing dental neurovascular bundle
11 Labial bone of Mandible
12 Concavities of the roots
13 Areolar bone surrounding the teeth
14 Unerupted (Wisdom tooth) = M3
15 Gomphosis = tooth/bone joint

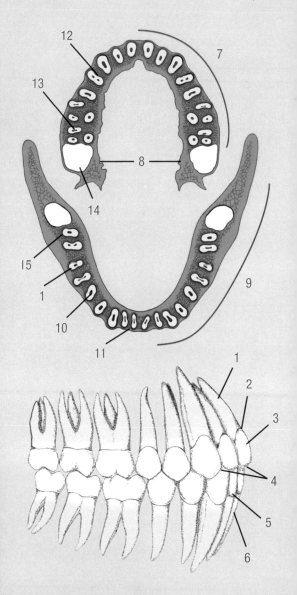

A **Teeth – Tooth types -**

B **Incisor**

C **Premolar 2 roots** (a molar would have 3 roots)

D *Longitudinal*

E 1 Enamel = substantia adamantine

F 2 Dentine = dentin

G 3 Gingival epithelium – covering the gum

H 4 Gum = gingiva

I 5 Loose CT – vascular bone marrow

   6 Cementum

J 7 Periodontum – strong fibrous vascular CT

K   (containing fibres of Cementum)

L 8 Alveolar bone*

M 9 Root canal continuous with the pulp = central cavity
    of the tooth, and it goes to the root foramen to allow

N   Ns and BVs to leave the tooth

O 10 Inferior dental N

P 11 Inferior dental v

Q 12 Inferior dental a

   13 10 + 11 + 12 = neurovascular bundle of the tooth

R 14 mental canal – base of the root foramen

S

*alveolar bone = air bone = bone with teeth embedded and "air" in b/n
T the spicules to lighten the jaw and act as shock absorbers.

U

V

W

X

Y

Z

© A. L. Ne

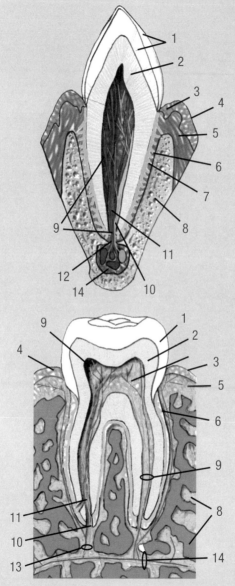

Temporo – Mandibular Joint = TMJ

closed - lateral / medial

open - sagittal

(only SYNOVIAL joint in the skull).

BS *superficial temporal & maxillary arteries*

NS *auriculotemporal & masseteric branches of mandibular branch of Trigeminal N (CN V)*

A *depression/elevation, protrusion/retraction, lateral movements*

1 Fibrous capsule

2 Lateral TMJ lig

3 Stylomandibular lig

4 Mandible

5 Ant. Temporal attachment of meniscus

6 Meniscus

7 Ant. mandibular attachment

8 Condyle of mandible

9 Posterior attachment

10 Sphenomandibular lig

11 Posterior temporal attachment

12 Lower joint compartment

13 Temporal bone

14 Upper compartment

15 Ext. auditory meatus

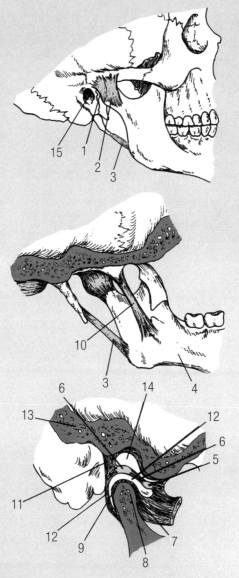

15 1 2 3

10

3 14 4

6 14 12

13 6 5

11

12 9 8 7

A
Tongue – in situ

B
Superior – looking onto its dorsal surface

C
Description: The tongue is "a bag of highly mobile skeletal muscle"
D
– one of the strongest muscles in the body, covered with a tough
stratified epithelium in which specialized epithelial structures are
E
inserted – the taste buds AKA papillae, along with mucous glands.

F
1   Epiglottis

G
2   median glossoepiglottic fold

3   epiglottic vallecula – crevice

H
4   root of the tongue - posterior1/3 – immobile part of
I
    the tongue

J
5   palatopharyngeus

6   palatine tonsil

K
7   palatoglossus

L
8   triangular fold

9   palatoglossal arch

M
10 median sulcus

N
11 dorsum of the tongue – pre-sulcus

O
12 margin of the tongue

13 body

P
14 tip of tongue = apex

Q
15 site of filiform papillae

R
16 fungiform papillae

17 folate papillae

S
18 circumvallate papillae

T
19 dorsum of the tongue – post-sulcus

U
20 sulcus terminalis

21 tonsilar fossa & crypts

V
22 foramen caecum

W
23 lingual tonsils –on the root/base of the tongue

X
24 lateral glossoepiglottic fold

Y
Taste buds – described based upon their shape – morphology see
Z
tongue surface and tastebuds.

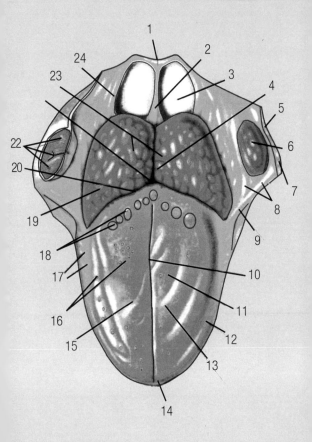

Tongue – in situ

Coronal – 2 sections through the tongue anteriorly
                    posteriorly (prior to the root of the tongue)

Description: The tongue is "a bag of highly mobile skeletal muscle" - one of the strongest muscles in the body. The anterior 2/3 mobile part of the tongue has several muscles arranged across all planes for maximum flexibility and adaptability to serve both for digestion and articulation.

1   median sulcus

2   vertical linguali m

3   transverse linguali m

4   sublingual fold

5   frenulum

6   inf mucosa of the tongue

7   ant sublingual salivary glands

8   epithelial covering of the tongue

9   midline raphe + lingual septum

10 longitudinal lingual i = inf. / s = superior

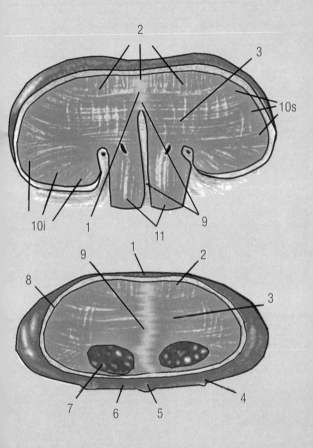

A
Tongue – in situ

B
Sagittal – looking into its middle surface

C
Description: The tongue is "a bag of highly mobile skeletal muscle" – one of the strongest muscles in the body. The anterior 2/3 mobile part of the tongue has several muscles arranged across all planes for maximum flexibility and adaptability to serve both for digestion and articulation.

1 Epiglottis

2 median glossoepiglottic fold

3 Vallecula of the epiglottis (space)

4 Root of the tongue – posterior 1/3 - immobile part of the tongue

5 Lingual tonsils – on the root/base of the tongue

6 Foramen caecum

7 Lingual septum

8 Transverse linguali m

9 Vertical linguali m

10 Basement Membrane

11 Epithelial lining of the tongue / mucosa of the tongue

12 Dorsum of the tongue – pre-sulcus + Tooth incisor

13 lower lip – muscles of facial expression in the fascia of this tissue

14 Buccal vestibule

15 Lingual vestibule + Frenulum

16 Mandible

17 Genioglossus m

18 Mylohyoid m

19 Geniohyoid m

20 subcutaneous fat

21 Hyoid

22 Laryngeal cartilage

23 Laryngeal ventricle

24 Larynx – superior aperture

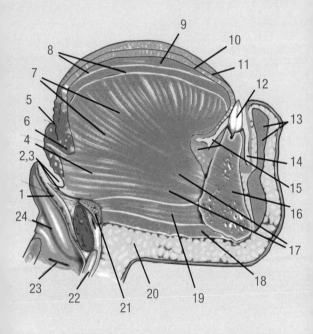

A # **Tongue – in situ**

B *Lateral – looking onto its lateral side – side of face removed*

C **Description:** The tongue is "a bag of highly mobile skeletal
D muscle" – controlled by a number of Ns – one for special senses
  – taste as well as innervation of its many muscles to serve both
E for digestion and articulation, eating and speaking.

F 1 Chorda Tympani from CN VII

G 2 Lingual N from CN V$_3$ + submandibular ganglion

  3 Tongue

H 4 Mandible

I 5 Frenulum + lingual vestibule

J 6 Mylohyoid m

K 7 Hypoglossus m

L 8 Deep lingual v

M 9 Hyoid bone

  10 Dorsal lingual a

N 11 Lingual a

O 12 Ext. carotid art + internal jugular v

P 13 Hypoglossal N (CN XII)

Q 14 Stylogossus m

R 15 Glossopharyngeal N (CN IX)

S 16 Mastoid process + Styloid process

T 17 Superior pharyngeal constrictor m

U

V

W

X

Y

Z

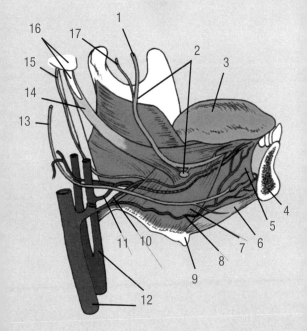

Tongue papillae + Taste bud

Schematic Tongue papilla – sagittal section
Schematic detailed cellular view of the taste bud.

Description: The tongue is a triangular muscle which is free and pointy at the at the distal end the Apex but which widens and is fixed at the proximal end - the Root. Although specialized structures sensitive to taste are found throughout the tongue's surface, taste buds - they are concentrated in the root of the tongue where they line the papillae. Ns attach to these "taste buds" which convey their information via CN V_3. At this point the lingual tonsilar material is also concentrated, as part of the tonsilar ring of defense at the entrance to the oropharynx

1 Circumvallate papilla
2 Filiform papilla
3 Mucosa
4 Lymphoid tissue
5 Crypt
6 Salivary gland
7 Tastebuds – N endings in the papillary crypts
8 Skeletal muscle
9 Stratified epithelium – on the tongue's surface carried into the crypts - near the taste buds
10 Taste pore
11 Taste villi
12 Taste cells
13 N filaments
14 Sustenacular cells – for support

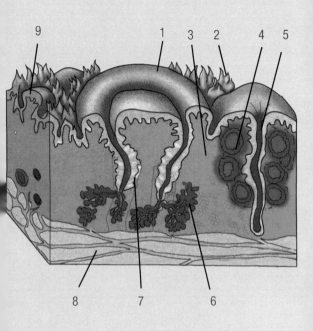

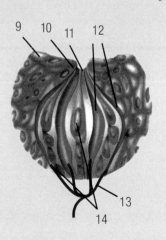

A
Transverse Colon – variations

B *Description:* the Transverse colon AKA the Horizontal colon lies b/n
C the ascending and the descending colon – from the hepatic flexure
to the splenic flexure. It has its own mesentery and is not fixed to
D the posterior abdominal wall, unlike the other 2 segments, it can
E vary in length and accounts for variations seen on Xrays.

F   1   Hepatic flexure

G   2   Transverse colon

H   3   Splenic flexure

I

J

K

L

M

N

O

P

Q

R

S

T

U

V

W

X

Y

Z

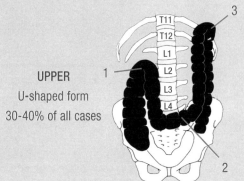

UPPER
U-shaped form
30-40% of all cases

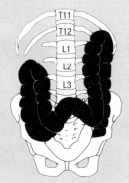

MIDDLE
W-shaped form
10-20% of all cases

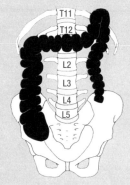

LOWER
stairway form
25% men /
10% women

A

Villi– of the Small Intestine

B   *Definition:* The SI has structured folds - the Plicae Circulares upon
C   which further increases in surface area is achieved via the Villi –
    protrusions of mucosa into the lumen.

D   Each villous contains a line of simple epithelium which to further
E   maximise the surface area for nutrient absorption has protrusions
    of cytoplasm on their surface the Microvilli.

F
    These cells divide at the base and move to the tip before being
G   sloughed every 3 days.

H
    A = small intestine

I   B = villi

J   C = intestinal epithelium

K   1   Surface epithelial cells – columnar

L   2   Microvilli on each cell for better absorption

M   3   Lamina Propria = loose CT filled with BVs, Ns,
        lymphoid tissue and monocytes
N
    4   Goblet cell – spills its cytoplasm in the lumen to
O   lubricate the contents of the SI

P   5   Younger epithelial cell – moving towards the tip

Q   6   Venous – blood going to the portal system - LP and
        slow flowing – full of nutrients
R
    7   Lacteal – specialized lymphatic of the SI
S
    8   Arterial supply to the villous
T
    9   Basal cells
U

V

W

X

Y

Z

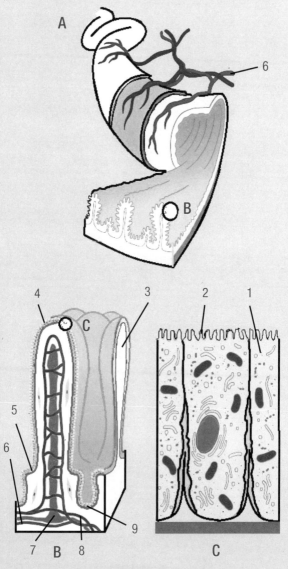

A

B

C

6

4 C 3 2 1

5

6

9

7 B 8 C

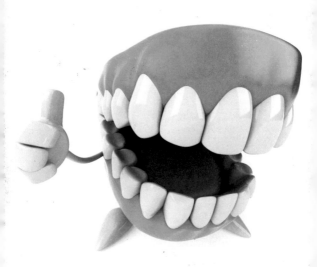